INCREASING VALUE

Sarah

Best Wishes

Phil

"Commissioning is first and foremost about patients. Clinical commissioning is about how, as clinicians, we can do more for our patients and vastly extend the depth and range of the possible. It is the coming of age of frontline clinicians, who are now able to have a major impact on the health of the local population, as well as treating the individual patient in front of them.

Yet many frontline clinicians regard commissioning with suspicion. They hear about the politics, the disputes and the dilemmas. There is endless talk about boards, bureaucracy and budgets. It hardly seems the fulfilment of their dreams, or the means by which they can achieve the most extreme ambitions for their patients.

That is why Philip De Silva's book is so timely and important. It speaks to frontline clinicians in language and with values that they understand. The author is not only a dedicated and expert commissioner, but also a first class communicator at the peak of his art.

In his preface he asks the question "How do frontline professionals survive the destruction and uncertainty of NHS reorganisation?" The answer lies in this book. It is to become a vital and effective cog in that reorganisation and for clinicians to lead it. This book will show you how to do that and how as a clinical community we might overcome those problems that pose the greatest threats to our patients:- whether it be lack of resources or a crisis of caring. This book is not simply for clinicians with an interest in commissioning. This book should be read by every frontline clinician".

Dr. Michael Dixon OBE, is a GP in Cullompton and Chair of the NHS Alliance.

Increasing Value is an excellent place to start for those new to the Commissioning agenda, whether clinicians or managers, and offers very practical insights into real and pervasive problems across the NHS, supported by a series of case studies.

The publication addresses fundamental questions all those involved in the commissioning process need to ask themselves , including how and where to invest finite resources to maximise value for populations. It explains programme budgeting in simple, clear terms, to enable commissioners to understand how to achieve greater benefit from shifting resources, toward greater identified need and offers a method of understanding spend, as well as how or where resources are allocated and what benefits they bring to a population.

At a time when much of primary care is focused on the shape of bureaucracies and organisations, *Increasing Value* stresses the importance of understanding population health needs and building local systems to address those needs, rather than the current focus on numbers and geography. It reminds us that the system of care, or the way the NHS collectively provides care for the public, is the driver for value and quality, rather than structures. We need to put more focus on the system we function in and imagine how good it could be if clinicians pulled together with managers to support change.

The publication also signposts very valuable tools and websites to aid commissioners in their ceaseless drive towards quality improvement; it offers suggestions on how to disinvest to fund appropriate innovations – a must in these times of economic challenge – through an understanding of the relation of spend to outcomes.

The approach adopted throughout *Increasing Value* is pragmatic and is based on a genuine understanding of the tensions and challenges facing all those working in the NHS. I particularly valued the section on embracing patient empowerment; one of the cornerstones of the commissioning agenda, if we are to be successful in our new role as commissioners, and I whole heartedly commend this publication to you.

Dr Johnny Marshall is Chairman of The National Association of Primary Care.

INCREASING VALUE

COMMISSIONING ON THE FRONT LINE

Philip DaSilva

With a Foreword by Dr. David Colin-Thome

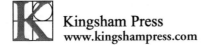

Kingsham Press
www.kingshampress.com

First published in 2012
by Kingsham Press

Oldbury Complex
Marsh Lane
Easthampnett
Chichester, West Sussex
PO18 0JW
United Kingdom

Typeset in Garamond

Printed and bound in the UK

ISBN: 978-1-904235-71-2

British Library Cataloging in Publication Data
A catalogue record of this book is available from the British Library

DaSilva, Philip

for Helen, Kate & Emma

ABOUT THE AUTHOR

Phil DaSilva has a nursing background and spent his clinical career driving a strong commitment to developing seamless care for patients across primary, secondary and community services. He has been successful in developing credible integrated clinical services, working with all professionals to ensure patients received the right care from the right professional at the right time.

Phil left clinical practice in 1994 to become Executive Director of Primary Care and Commissioning and has held other senior executive and national roles where he has been influential in the development of commissioning - through the era of GP fund-holding, the development and re-organisation of PCTs and the introduction of practice based commissioning. He has used his clinical understanding to retain a focus on patients, particularly during periods of upheaval and change. He was a successful PCT Chief Executive and is currently the joint leader of the National QIPP Right Care Programme.

Phil has a first class honours degree in Nursing, a Masters in Public Health and has written this book, in part, as preparation to study for a Doctorate. He is a trained Executive coach and the views in this book are entirely the author's, shared with front line professionals to encourage them to think about patients and population health during periods of change and to acknowledge the opportunities they have to engage in commissioning. He is the co-author of the *NHS Atlas of Variation*.

■
ACKNOWLEDGEMENTS

This book would not have been started, had I not received the encouragement of some but the support of many, to write and share my experiences and insights about clinicians connecting with the system to enhance commissioning.

The names of those who have helped shaped my career are too many to mention. Working with you all has been rewarding in every way; but particular thanks are due to Dennis, Chris, Mary, Cliff, Bob and Jean who have reminded me to keep a focus on the thing that matters - patients and improving their care – and of course, Muir, who has inspired and driven me to complete this book.

I also wish to thank those who have shared their experiences through coaching sessions and particularly to those who have shared their stories in this book. I'm sure you will recognise yourselves; thank you!

■
CONTENTS

FOREWORD

Dr. David Colin-Thome

Whatever emerges from changes to the landscape of the NHS, one thing seems certain - we need a fresh approach to commissioning. A big task and one we need to re-define without adding to its complexity by continuing to focus too much on the structures, size of organisations and its bureaucracy. Instead, we need to focus much more on the patient and populations health to improve outcomes.

Many commentators, internal and external to the NHS, identify an under achievement of NHS commissioning, and some of it with merit. The NHS in general and its commissioners in particular usually adopt a very hierarchical and often reductionist managerial approach. In a complex adaptive system such as the NHS, linear approaches to management are of limited value and effect, especially when it pertains to clinical commissioning. Effective commissioners need to exhibit clarity of purpose in a multiplicity of relationships within a complex system, with a focus on increasing value for the patients and population.

Clinical commissioning groups led by general medical practitioners, is a fresh opportunity for all clinicians to shape the system and encourage a better focus on outcomes and value for their patients. This can be achieved chiefly by focusing more on commissioning for individual patients as the essential building block for a population responsibility.

Clinical commissioners cannot function in splendid isolation and need to enlist providers in their task - working collaboratively, describing outcomes and not prescribing of processes. Relationships and power dynamics will need to therefore radically change so the individual provider organisation, not the commissioner, is clearly and explicitly accountable for its care quality and population focus. Clinically led commissioning can facilitate this by aligning their activity with budgetary responsibility. After all, it is those clinical leaders who too often are 'invisible' to the public gaze, yet it is they who 'spend' the money by their deployment of clinical resources.

Making hard decisions is a core commissioning task so clinical commissioners need to ensure both a public transparency and the public's effective involvement and engagement, to be the 'people's organisation'. To obtain commissioning support clinical commissioning groups must view themselves as the customer and need to identify a choice of support, maybe in conjunction with other groups.

A lot to ask but a necessary ask for commissioners to exhibit a leadership of a complex adaptive fiercely local system. A test writ large for a clinician leadership and an opportunity to slightly paraphrase, yet challenge the Dr Julian Tudor Hart aphorism 'clinicians often lay claim to ground they do not wish to occupy'[1].

A lot to ask, but a necessary ask, for the essential continued development of commissioning and more importantly, the role clinicians play in commissioning.

This timely book offers insights into the development of commissioning. It focuses the reader to remember the core business of the NHS is to improve patient care and increase value and presents concepts for all clinicians and managers alike, to consider to engage in the developing world of commissioning.

Dr David Colin-Thomé

Honorary visiting professor at Manchester Business School, Manchester University and of the School of Health, University of Durham

Former General Medical Practitioner at Castlefields Health Centre, Runcorn, England and National Clinical Director of Primary Care, Department of Health England

---

[1] Hart J. *A New Kind of Doctor. (1989)* Merlin Press.

PREFACE

At a time of organisational turmoil, it is sometimes easy to forget our patients. It is also too simple to create a divide between those clinicians delivering a service at the front-line, those responsible for planning or commissioning and those whose main role is to lead and manage the services. The reality should be that there is no division but rather, a greater integration of front-line professional expertise and knowledge to:

- improve care to patients
- inform the commissioning cycle
- increase value from resources.

The question has been asked so many times, sometimes from people with commissioning in their job title, as to:

- what is commissioning?
- who does it?
- how do commissioners know what we, at the front line, are doing and
- how do they know what works for our patients?
- is commissioning a management task or clinical role?

This book is a response to all those questions and many more. It presents an opportunity for clinicians and other front-line professionals, of all disciplines and grades to maintain a focus on delivering high quality care and to engage with the commissioning agenda, more so during times of upheaval, as it is at that time that patients may too easily be forgotten. This book will hopefully encourage many front-line professionals to make a wider contribution at improving health care for the whole population, as well as for their own patients, contributing to the commissioning of safe, effective and sustainable programmes of care.

The book will not make you an expert commissioner overnight, but is designed to prompt you to think how and where you can, perhaps already unknowingly do, contribute to the commissioning of care. It will raise some concepts, to help you, as front-line professionals to maximise value, whatever your position in the NHS.

Furthermore, it is neither a technical manual on "how to commission", nor is it written for the expert commissioner, although it will be of interest to that audience; rather, it is written with front-line clinicians and managers in mind to illustrate how – and more importantly why – they should engage in commissioning.

The material covered here aims to prompt readers to consider issues and seek out more information and resources on topics such as value, programme budgeting and variation. In highlighting these issues, it is hoped that front-line professionals will gain a deeper knowledge of commissioning and the confidence to engage for their patients and profession.

Increasing Value: Commissioning on the Front Line will also encourage readers to think differently about their own contribution to health care, beyond the excellent day to day care and support they provide, and to appreciate that commissioning is not, never has been, the protected domain of a few managers around the "top-table". All front-line professionals have a part to play, in contributing and supporting the people who are responsible for pulling it all together.

Key concepts discussed here are raised to engage with clinicians who have some managerial role, as well as managers who oversee clinicians. But there are tens of thousands of front line professional staff across primary care, community and acute settings including GPs, Practice Nurses, Health Visitors, District Nurses, Community Nurses, Consultants, Doctors, Ward Sisters, Physiotherapists, Occupational Therapists, other AHPs, Nurses, Laboratory Scientists, Pharmacists and a whole host of other professional groups, where the individual clinician is responsible for much more than their own time. This book is also for them as it embraces the process of maximising value from our resources. This begins with the allocation of you, your knowledge and skill as a resource to different patient groups in the process of commissioning and in providing commissioned care. It will involve considering which patients benefit the most from the resources to be allocated to them.

Of central importance in this book is the move away from the distraction of creating structures and new organisations, or focusing so heavily on institutions, health centres and hospitals as the basic unit of management of resources. The core businesses of healthcare are not confined only to institutions, notwithstanding the excellent care they provide. Our attention needs to be beyond the visible bricks and mortar. Problems like dementia, respiratory disease, diabetes, rheumatoid arthritis, pelvic pain, and mental health - are becoming key and testing issues of healthcare. This is why the model of a health service is one in which the institutions, which are necessary, are complemented by a set of programmes and systems; run by front-line professionals as an integrated system.

So, if you are thinking that it is the hospital, health centre or general medical practice which provides the care, the book will stimulate you to think beyond these buildings, introducing concepts which will enable you to consider the patient and their disease or condition rather than the institution. In doing so, it will enable us to think about the patient and systems around them and more importantly when commissioning services, on populations; to think about all the people with heart disease, diabetes, or with bipolar disorder – not just those who happen to have been referred to and identified within the service.

Finally, the book will offer some real life stories, anonymised of course, from coaching sessions. These will highlight how front-line professionals have managed themselves during periods of professional and organisational uncertainty, focussed on doing the right things, for the right patients and engaged in contributing to the wider health improvement agenda – integrating care.

INTRODUCTION

'Nurse, make sure you are with the right patient at the right time and not doing something for a patient that they can do for themselves – and when you are with those patients, make sure you do them no harm.'

Those words were spoken by Matron Cooke, during a meeting with cadet nurses in 1974. That time, incidentally, was similar to today as a period of significant reorganisation within the NHS, when the NHS Reorganisation Act July 1973, produced in 1972, by Sir Keith Joseph and the Conservative government, was implemented by Barbara Castle and the incoming Labour administration of 1974, (Gabe 1991, Klien 2006).

Successive governments have since declared the structure or management of the NHS to be unaffordable or not fit for purpose at that point. Re-organisations have happened frequently—with at least 15 identifiable major structural changes in three decades, as pointed out by Walshe (2010). Moreover, there has been a constant theme throughout; **it often feels as though more focus and energy goes into the reorganisation and development of new structures and bureaucracies than into designing, improving, efficient integrated patient care.**

The turmoil of reorganisation is a constant but necessary theme in a progressive NHS – not for reorganisation's sake, but to meet the ever rising demands, delivering innovative practice and introducing ever improving technology. We now face this challenge when investment is tight and the NHS needs to extract more value from its resources, beyond the tremendous improvements in healthcare which includes some fantastic innovations. That fact of the matter is that we still face significant challenges to make the NHS world class in all areas.

There have been wonderful advances in the detection and management of cancer; we know more about managing heart disease, stroke and diabetes; and we have improved interventions requiring surgery – including reducing the time patients need to spend in hospital following many operations. On the other hand, we are still seeing significant variance in services and in access to high quality care, and are now beginning to identify more unwarranted inconsistencies within the NHS. The concern is that these may not be addressed if managers and clinicians focus only on administrative reorganisations, rather than on enhancing the experience for patients and populations; improving outcomes through integrated clinical systems and care beyond the boundaries of organisations. Let us remember that patients and their carers remain in the middle of the reorganisation and churn and their needs must always come first.

The duty clinicians and other front line professionals hold to make this a reality is critical. The NHS can truly be world class if all disciplines, collectively draw on the positive spirit and focus that clinicians and managers alike put into managing organisational change and instead channel that joint commitment and improvement towards designing the systems and networks, and engaging with our patients. This book acknowledges some of the dilemmas they face in trying to achieve these whilst maintaining a safe service, put patients first and engage in commissioning, more so whilst it feels that there is too much to do!

The current proposed changes are again significant. They will alter the organisational structure by phasing out Strategic Health Authorities and Primary Care Trusts by 2013, and creating new Clinical Commissioning Groups to be accountable for the majority of the NHS budget, to commission services for their population. Furthermore, given historical trends, this is unlikely to be the last re-organisation of the NHS. So, how do front-line professionals survive the distraction and uncertainty of the current or for that matter other reorganisation of the NHS?

The words of Matron Cooke and many other senior clinicians and managers have shaped the way many professionals have worked. In essence, they maintained a fundamental belief that we are here in the NHS to serve the needs of patients, carers and the public before the needs, even ambitions, of organisations, clinicians or managers.

This book is designed to help clinicians and managers in all roles, and at all levels of practice, in all organisations, to remember what it was that brought them into the NHS and why they do what they do. Patient care and the improvement of the health of the population is the optimal and ultimate goal. The book offers ways to help retain this focus during periods of enormous upheaval, introducing new concepts to help address the challenge that yet more structural turmoil may bring.

The intention is to help professionals sustain a focus on the patient and the care they provide. The book aims to stimulate readers to look more widely and think differently when they consider what they do today for their patients. An essential starting point is for us all to ask ourselves a few questions as follows:.

- What am I trying to achieve with the resources available?
- What budgets am I using?
- How does the quality and volume of care I provide compare with others?
- What is the system I work in?
- What role do I play in maintaining the efficiency of that system?
- Am I seeing the right patient?
- Do I have any responsibility for population health beyond the patient in front of me?
- Are there patients not being seen who should be?
- Could this patient be treated better in a different environment?
- Am I providing added value to the treatment of this patient?

1

INCREASING NEED, RISING DEMAND, AND NO MORE MONEY

'Increasing need, rising demand, and no more money – what the hell are we going to do?

Obiter dicta

I n every society and across the world, this profound call is repeated because whilst the NHS in England is a unique institution, it is not alone in the challenges it faces. Every health service will have to meet increasing need and demand rising faster than the increase in resources. So, what can be done?

Well, often staff are asked to do more but with little explanation as to why, or more importantly, how! So whilst the call to 'work harder' has been a traditional approach, it is of limited appeal to a workforce that is already working flat out, at coping with new ways of working and increasing demands. 'Work smarter' is a more modern slogan and it is essential to ensure that health services improve quality, that they do things better, safer, cheaper and without duplication or waste, so that care is provided using as few, but the right, resources; both financial and individual, as possible. Again, these measures are necessary but not sufficient to meet the challenges of the future.

What is needed is not just to do things better or differently, but to do the right things – to do the right things right, but to use the old management proverb – what is meant by *the right things to do?*

The NHS and Commissioning

The development of clinical commissioning needs to be considered with a fresh approach and be a change from the current process driven model of commissioning. The future must be different, but it is not good enough to simply expect all clinicians to turn their minds to commissioning. It needs thought and imagination. Many Primary Care Trusts have demonstrated excellent and innovative ways of engaging, capturing and extending clinical input to the commissioning cycle, but it is not standard good practice everywhere.

Managers and clinicians need to come closer together, consider and share the benefit of this increasing clinical input. The future is not a place waiting for our arrival, like Everest or the Great Barrier Reef; it is something that is imagined, planned and created.

It is the same for clinical commissioning; we need to imagine it, build it and ensure it becomes the business of all clinicians and their front-line professional colleagues engaging with the health improvement agenda. If we do not imagine, plan and build a new model of commissioning, then the fresh opportunity to place clinicians at the centre of commissioning may be lost and usurped by others, not by managers stepping forward, but clinicians stepping backwards, perhaps to avoid the role conflict they fear of becoming a hybrid manager (Lewis, 2001). It is vital that as the new world is being imagined and built that clinicians are supported, developed and encouraged to engage and contribute.

The opportunity is here and now, what some have referred to as a pivotal point in the history of our nation and the NHS. Not only are we observing new political arrangements by the first peacetime Coalition government since the 1930s, but we are also at a crossroads in British society, as a result of the serious economic downturn within which we are having to refocus the NHS (Easton, 2011). When fused together, these herald a new dawning for the NHS in England, where dramatic and significant changes are being proposed. In themselves, they create opportunities in our healthcare system, opportunities for greater clinical leadership, which is both necessary and achievable. The drive to develop clinical leadership is not new. There are good descriptions of some of the definitions, barriers and opportunities (Stanton *et al* 2010).

Commissioning is not new either and Commissioners have become more agile over recent years, moving well away from an approach based on, say, transactional management of contracts with primary or secondary care institutions in a transactional process, to one which is becoming more transformational, with wider partnership arrangements to improve health and well-being. However, the term commissioning has been used to describe many things, confounded and mystified by departments and bureaucracies. This chapter will offer some insights into commissioning and how clinicians at all levels can, some would argue should, get more involved.

Commissioning or CO-Mission-ing?

What is commissioning? How does it work and how do we know what patients need? These are very challenging questions, ones which cannot be addressed fully in this book. However, there are some key principles to dissect, to understand how commissioning can deliver improvements in the health of individual patients and wider populations – and why clinicians, with their patients, should be at the forefront of this process.

The first principle to remember is that commissioning for health and well- being is underpinned by patient needs not wants. There is no real end point to effective commissioning; it is a cycle of change and improvement.

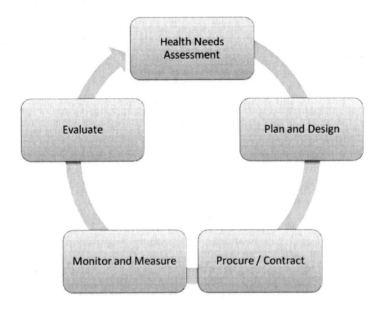

FIGURE 1:THE COMMISSIONING CYCLE

To offer some insight into the domain of commissioning, this book will refer to a clinician who has helped to de-mystify the process of commissioning so as to retain the focus on patients.

Dr Peter Brambleby helpfully reminded us all that the "mission" is at the heart of it. To say it slowly as ... *"co – mission – ing"* describes it easily! He goes on to describe it thus:

- The "co-" i.e the prefix reminds us of the interdependence between the parties.
- The "-mission-" in the middle reminds us of the need for common purpose.
- The "-ing" i.e the suffix reminds us that this is a verb; an active process that takes the local NHS to a different place by doing something. (Brambleby 2010)

At the very centre is the mission, and the mission is to improve health, relieve distress and disability, close the gap on avoidable inequalities, and achieve all that within a given budget.

To "commission" is, therefore, to unite the interested parties around a common purpose and a shared understanding of resources – not just money – to increase value and improve quality.

Value, a concept which is discussed later, is about improving quality and delivering safe effective care with an awareness of its cost. To "add value" requires a constant appraisal and reappraisal of the return on the investment that is being made in healthcare services. It means systematically reviewing services and systems and making transparent decisions to stop doing those things of lower value, in favour of those with higher value. This demands added impetus, using clinical skills and determination when resources are tight or shrinking. It requires all interested parties and particularly clinicians to take the lead and work together integrating the health system, reaching greater consensus to identify and deliver higher value interventions and better outcomes.

It can be argued that the commissioning arena has lacked the contribution and engagement of front line professionals to provide some of the information and knowledge of the population's needs. Until now, it has been predominately managers, some with a clinical background and organisations, both within and outside NHS, which have taken centre stage in identifying local needs and more importantly providing shape to that service. Strong and supported clinical leadership will be critical to engage all parties with the commissioning cycle, if it is to succeed in increasing value, improving quality and delivering a safe and effective NHS.

Moreover, the positive shift away from a narrow focus on contracting from a primary and/or secondary care perspective, towards a much more inclusive and wider perspective is welcomed. Again this needs to involve front-line professionals, health and social care working with education, third sector and the population.

Clinical Commissioning Groups must be supported to build this approach if they are to become fully engaged, embracing this fresh opportunity, and moving the NHS away from inputs and outputs, to one which can demonstrate better outcomes and maximise value for the population served from the resources invested. The focus will then be on the money spent on a service and its outcomes – the value achieved from that resource. The responsibility for clinicians to understand their contribution is the key – particularly in analysing variations in access, activity, spend and outcomes. The responsibility for the NHS is to ensure those clinicians are supported and helped to make the change. In this way, opportunities can be identified to increase value, enhance quality and reduce unwarranted variation.

The interested parties in added value are:

- the recipients of care
- the providers of care
- those who hold the funds
- those who set policy and strategy
- the research community who provide evidence and evaluation.

Ask yourself:

Which are the key parties in your system?
What is your contribution to their care?
How do you link with others in your system to share knowledge?
How could you strengthen and make better use of those links?

These are key challenges for any reorganisation. So how can the NHS respond? **Well, first we must acknowledge that the change offers opportunities to put clinicians in the commissioning driving seat – a real opportunity for front-line professionals, not just general practitioners, to engage with specialist clinicians from the secondary care sector.** But how is it possible to understand the true needs of the population and prioritise services accordingly? Crucially, a fuller understanding will prevent all resources being devoted only to those with known demands. Knowledge of the needs of population will also avoid following a historical path of providing the same services without any focus or redesign, doing what has always been done, bringing the same results, as Berwick (1996) so eloquently has commented *"every system is perfectly designed to get the results it gets"*. We need to embrace change for our patients and to get best value from our resources.

There are tools to help clinician's understand and appreciate how and where to allocate resources. **The first tool is programme budgeting, with its related discipline of marginal analysis.** This offers a way of simplifying the challenge by understanding expenditure by disease group, then using that expenditure as a fixed point to start discussions about improving health and increasing value. How many times have clinicians claimed that "if only we had more resource" or "we need to make some investment" in our service, without fully appreciating the level of investment currently made and how that resource is allocated and what outcomes are delivered?

And so the starting point here is for every clinician and for that matter health care professional to reflect upon, analyse and discuss key questions as follows:

- How much do you spend in the service that you and your team provides? If you don't know, who should you be asking for such data?
- Apart from what you spend on the service which you and your team provides, what is the "actual cost" of the service that you and your team provides?
- What added value can you think of that can be derived from re-allocating any of that resource to an alternative process to improve patient outcomes?
- What is the value of your service?
- What waste, if any can you think of in the system in which you function? What can be stopped, safely, to release resource to other areas of clinical practice?

"Programme budgeting" is a technique for describing where the money in a local health system, such as a PCT, has been deployed. This is broken down into manageable and meaningful programmes related to objectives, with the intention of tracking and influencing future deployment of programme resources. Programme budgeting has its critics, but serious application of programme budgeting is well beyond infancy in the NHS and more and more PCTs and commissioners have realised its potential and it is now gaining more credibility, as definitions are agreed, Tsourapas A (2011).

"Programmes" are defined to meet the planning and operational needs of the service. They might be disease groups, age groups, geographical locations or settings for care, to name a few. They can also be constructed as a matrix so that, for example, a set of disease-based programmes could also be broken down by provider or age group. To illustrate, we will use an example of Tweetshire PCTs Programme Budget spend for Respiratory Care:

Take a look at the grid below and work out a process for agreeing where spend should be allocated? Should respiratory spend stay at its current £75 million an increase of 5% per year in Tweetshire? Do we know how much we should be allocating to respiratory conditions – what is the need? Going through each of these phases, asking questions to understand how the allocation to a single disease can be understood within that disease category or group, not simply as a single disease, but broken down into smaller sections, can be most illuminating.

To take this a bit further, allocate in phase three for instance, what you consider to be the right level of investment and work out how you would be able to do this? To illustrate, let us take a slice of the programme budgeting spend for Tweetshire and from the top three conditions focus on one to understand how it can be broken down into a workable programme; we will use respiratory care as an example here but you can use the model for other conditions.

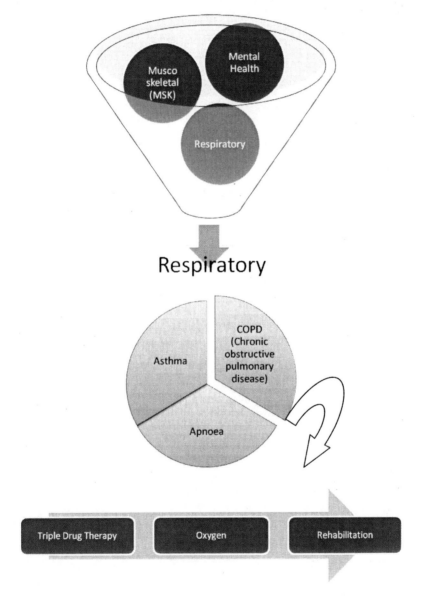

FIGURE 2: PROGRAMME BUDGETING EXERCISE: INTRA-SYSTEM MARGINAL ANALYSIS
(produced with permission- Gray 2011)

So, using the model to think about the care you provide, or commission, can you determine how much money is currently going into that system? Use the model to understand how the money is both *allocated* and *utilised*. Where do you think the money could best be directed to improve care and outcomes for your patients? It's not a simple exercise, but once understood it can illuminate the way systems are developed and funded. Some can appear large whilst others appear less funded, thus creating a distortion to care. By doing this clinicians, can start to understand some of the opportunities commissioning offers them to direct resources to areas of greater benefit.

Below is an opportunity to have a go in Tweetshire:

Table 1: Modelling of Current Spend on Respiratory Conditions

Phase 1 Current spend by programme budget for respiratory conditions in local town CCG is £75m

Programme	Population	Clinical commissioning group	Current Spend	Planned Spend
Respiratory	Tweetshire PCT	Local town	£75 million	£ ? million

Phase 2 The Programme budget broken down into smaller workable conditions

Programme	Population	Applied to	Allocation by condition	Spend
Respiratory	Local town	COPD	£40 million	
	Clinical commissioning group	Sleep apnoea	£5 million	£75 million
		Asthma	£30 million	

Phase 3 Allocate your resources to the areas of this condition

Programme	Population	System	Planned Allocation by condition	Actual Spend Spend
Your Programme				

This offers a way to think differently about how much resource is targeted at a condition and the importance of a sound understanding of the health needs of that population. Without it, resources may be allocated unfairly or based on historical activity and uptake. The important issue to remember is that the investment can only be used once and it should be directed to gain the greatest benefit for the population. Clinicians are central to that allocation process. They understand the condition and see the benefits of the investment through their patients; they also see the waste and duplication which should be eradicated to increase value.

Reform: A fresh opportunity for Clinicians?

The NHS principles from 1948 to the present day have been underpinned by fairness, being free at the point of delivery and availability for those in need, McBride *et al*, (2010). The NHS reforms have reinforced this philosophy, but it is being challenged at a time when significant savings will need to be made from the NHS to reinvest in future health care, Appleby *et al*, (2010).

The sentiment behind the launch of the White Paper, *Equity and Excellence: Liberating the NHS*, (Department of Health, 2010) has generated many comments, (both positive and negative) about its boldness, ambition and pace. The manner in which current health reform unfolds will be shaped by some, influenced by many and commented on by even more. Perhaps, it is worth noting that the same had been claimed in previous reorganisations, regardless of the political shade of government, where similar reforms attempted to promote clinicians to play a key role in the planning and delivery of care.

That being said however, it is crucial to ask what role can clinicians have in shaping the change to ensure the NHS mantra of doing the right things for the right patients? Well, one certainty is that the redesign of services and system reform must not be left to managers and Executive Boards alone. It must involve patients and clinicians to a much greater extent than has been the case for many years, appealing to clinicians at all levels – with a focus on building systems, increasing value and engaging patients to plan, design and deliver effective care.

However, the knowledge base for effective interventions is dauntingly large and sometimes overwhelming for practicing clinicians. It can be used as a defence and a block to action or reform. The data, some of which may even appear contradictory, can cover every stage of the patient pathway from prevention to end-of-life support. There may be evidence to weigh up for all the intervening steps along the way, such as diagnostics, treatments and continuing care. However, the skilled practitioner must be able to use these data sources to create knowledge and apply evidence to support the investments required – not only for the patient alongside them, but also to meet the identified and continued needs of the wider population and future patients.

This balance is a constant challenge to commissioners to ensure services are available and delivered in a safe, clinically and cost effective way. Currently, Primary Care Trusts hold the responsibility for commissioning care for their population, but this is changing rapidly, as the responsibility for a majority of commissioning passes to clinical commissioning groups. There is, yet again, an inherent danger that the service will focus on the organisation and structure of the commissioning groups or the bureaucracy wrapped around them, rather than the systems required to deliver high value care. A most important issue here is the support and development of clinicians to understand their responsibilities of the new commissioning arrangements and the important role they play.

So, whilst the organisation and bureaucracy is important, we must also pay attention to the opportunities patients and clinicians alike have to seize the initiative and redefine the NHS as a system to meet the needs of its population and patients, with supporting organisations and bureaucracies behind that system.

In building new systems, a recurring question many clinicians ask is, "why have we got some of the organisational challenges we currently experience?" Beyond re-organisation, what can be done to ameliorate or even avoid them in future planning?. Maybe the simple answer is that if we were starting from scratch, the NHS would perhaps look very different; we would stop doing some things and start doing others; we would have services in different parts of the system and we might even have more effective remote technology to break the dependency culture on hospital care that we have in today's NHS.

The reality is that the NHS is overwhelmed with history and emotional attachment and it is not quite as simple as is being talked about to make the changes necessary. We all have at least one view on how much money and where resources should be allocated or changed. Fisher (2007) describes how resource allocation within the NHS, has been a fascinating lesson of debates about who should set and manage the priorities, and the arguments about heuristics and values. It will be valuable for us all to acquaint ourselves with some of those insights.

However, before moving the reader to consider new concepts, it is useful to look back and reflect on previous reorganisations to appreciate that we should place as much energy in developing systems and patient services, when putting front line clinicians in charge as we do when making changes to the architectures.

The Past

The NHS formed in 1948 spent its first ten years focused on disease and the eradication of some of the big killers such as TB, measles, cholera, and other infectious diseases. The following two decades focused on treatment and prevention, probably in that order, with the NHS enjoying times of rapid growth and development. Since then there have been the technological and information revolutions and the switch to "market forces" (albeit a managed market). Now, in the 21st century we face a new challenge, intensified by the economic situation – namely, reconciling quality and value.

What can clinicians do to help shape the NHS? It is understandable that many clinicians will either not wish to understand structural reforms or be disinterested in the management and political agenda. However, in order to keep a focus on the patient and population's health, it is worth looking through the rear view mirror to see where we have come from and to see how these changes do in effect offer clinicians opportunities to lead. Structural change is a constant, where front-line clinicians are not only expected to continue to provide excellent care, but also to maintain a high quality service whilst others are preoccupied by the shifting deck chairs.

The NHS was initially organised around three components – hospitals, primary care, and local authority health services – and the reform in 1974 saw a 'unified' structure introduced at Regional, Area and District level. The number of bodies changed. Fourteen Regional Health Authorities, covering all three parts of the NHS and incorporating the teaching hospitals, replaced the previous authorities. This reorganisation was underpinned by consensus management and a belief that in a multidisciplinary NHS, all skill groups could have a voice in decisions. But the system was complex and managerially driven; it earned much criticism. So, can history really tell us what the system could have look like?

Let us examine an earlier interim report on the future provision of services. The report outlines the NHS as promoting primary and secondary care services. It offers some models of care and prescribed for:

- services designed around small primary care units;
- a supply chain to a hospital;
- a relationship with that hospital and medical schools;
- and specialist tertiary centres covering a wider geography.

If this sounds familiar, read on. The report commented on:

- The urgency for the orderly building of a constructive health policy, and the close relationship which needs to exist between **medical services and the problems connected with local government.**
- The general availability of medical services can only be effectively distributed according to the needs of the community. **This organisation is needed on grounds of efficiency and cost.**
- **Preventive and curative medicine cannot be separated** and must be brought together in close co-ordination.
- Primary health care should be based on secondary health care but all those **cases requiring special treatment could be referred** to, by and from primary care centres.
- **The equipment and support of the secondary care centres would be more extensive and the medical personnel more specialised.**
- Secondary care centres must (of necessity) be situated in towns with an efficient consultant service and adequate equipment. **These secondary care centres would vary in size** and elaboration according to circumstances.
- Primary health centres would often serve a much wider area and require special staff. They would comprise **provision for patients suffering from such conditions as tuberculosis, mental disease, epilepsy, certain infectious diseases, and those in need of orthopaedic treatment.**

The final statement should alert the reader to the fact that this not a new report. In fact, it was drafted by the then Health Minister, the Rt. Hon. Christopher Addison in 1920 and is possibly the first recording of the term primary care, in an official white paper (Starfield, *et al* 2005).

The report goes on to conclude that:

- "A primary health care centre, with its organised services **established by local enterprise**, will service its community well if it is conceived in the right spirit, put in the right place, and organised on the right lines.
- The services of the secondary health centre would be mainly of a consultative type. The centres would receive cases referred to them by primary care, either on account of **difficulties of diagnosis** or because in their diagnosis or treatment a higher **specialist equipment** was needful.
- Cases referred for consultation or treatment would attend at out-patient clinics, or would occupy in-patient beds in a secondary care centre, but every facility would be **afforded for general practitioners to keep in touch with their patients and to resume their medical supervision immediately on discharge**".

In sharing this report, it is worth reflecting on other significant health reports for two reasons. The first is to ask what we have been doing for nearly a hundred years and does the structure really play a bigger part than the system of care or the culture of the service? The second, is to illustrate that we have been trying to get the structures right, well before the birth of the NHS and that we may be in danger of missing the opportunity as we imagine, plan and build clinical commissioning. How will professionals ensure that territorial disputes around buildings and organisations do not dilute the effort and energy to design an integrated system of care? These questions are raised here, as it is of concern that there is frequently more commentary on the shape, size and geography of developing structures and far less on, say, identifying the number of diabetics in the population and what services they require – or the level of investment required to improve outcomes of planned respiratory care for a given population, regardless of organisation.

This is really where **clinical commissioning can play a significant part and take the lead in shaping services for our patients and populations. There is a great opportunity to engage clinicians and to carefully consider, imagine and build the supporting structures required to deliver high quality services which increase value, rather than what, say, primary care or secondary care can do in isolation.** After all, that will only retain the increasing dependence on the current commissioning cycle and behaviours and the dependence the NHS places on hospital care, which has to be reduced to increase value and meet rising demand with limited with resources.

The issue of value will be considered in more detail in the following chapter. But in a general sense, we should reflect on some of the language issues here. We should reflect and focus more on words such as 'patients' and 'populations' and reduce emphasis on words such as primary, community and secondary care. The latter refer to the organisations and buildings and maintain their dependence. It is better to place the focus on the patient and which part of the pathway of care is delivered best, by whom – in which environment to increase value.

Ten questions to consider:

1. Do you know how much your service spends now?
2. What outcomes are your population experiencing from this investment?
3. Do you understand how the £x million is allocated and distributed across, say, prescribing, out-patient activity, hospital admissions, your time and development etc?
4. How should such allocation change across the conditions?
5. Can resource be released by changing current practice?
6. Who is responsible for the utilisation of this resource?
7. Who is responsible and accountable for the design and allocation of resources for respiratory care?
8. Who is the lead clinician, ie who is "in charge"?
9. What service would the population like to see, for example, less unnecessary outpatient appointments or visits to hospital?
10. How can the patients and carers be involved in designing and evaluating the system?

Perhaps the eleventh and most important question should be "Why don't we know?"

2

INCREASING VALUE – DOING THE RIGHT THINGS & DOING THEM RIGHT

T he NHS can be usually be summed up in one word at any point in time. From its inception in 1948 until the publication of Cochrane's book *Effectiveness and Efficiency* in 1972, (Gray 2011) that word was 'free'. From about 1974 and through the 80's, the buzz word had been 'effective'; and for the rest of the 1990s, cost-effectiveness became the key word as concerns about resources started to multiply. In a positive move, from the turn of the century into 2000, the key word has been 'quality' and perhaps into 2012 and beyond the word may well be **"Value."**

For the past twenty years the concept of quality has been the key word for clinicians working with managers to create a safe and effective environment for patients. During this time we have seen the introduction of quality initiatives covering all aspects of care. But, Robert H Brook (2010), argues that *'after 40 years of academic analysis of quality improvement in healthcare, it is unclear what it has accomplished'*. Brook adds that *'In considering the next 50 years of quality assurance activities, what is needed is a health care system at the intersection of higher quality and lower cost.'*

These are the very matters which clinicians can influence the most:

- Doing the right thing for the right patient
- Influencing commissioning so that resources are allocated to higher value interventions
- Reducing duplication and eliminating waste
- Improving the population's health

This may sound a significant challenge. However, experience can demonstrate that clinicians want to engage but sometimes feel disempowered by managers or "commissioners". Let us explore this issue further, with a real short case study in in mind.

COACH A

Coach A: a skilled and experienced nurse who was leading a small respiratory team. The issue A found most difficult was why "the management" expected her to maintain so many different records for the patients she saw. On examination it was soon apparent that A was feeding information to many different organisations, often required in different format, with little understanding as to why. A realised that working close to a geographical boundary of two PCTs, she was expected to maintain care notes to meet the various organisations' need and risk registers – not the patients, family and her colleagues professional needs.

We explored what opportunities there were for making a change and whether A had raised this as an issue with anybody within the PCT or her line manager. Unfortunately, she did not know where to start or who to speak to. There was a history of tolerating behaviour rather than a pro- active approach.

Over a period of weeks, A realised that there was a possible solution but that nothing would change if she was not proactive. Inertia was not the issue, because A really wanted to do something to release time to care for her patients; the issue was that she did not feel empowered to do anything.

Over a period of months of working together, A did take action, changed the recording and paperwork (although sadly the two neighbouring organisations wanted their own and could not see why they should adopt the new patient recording logs!) and from many different forms and documents the respiratory service e, led by A, designed their own which kept all patients and clinicians informed and improved patient satisfaction and experience.

This was a small action but a big step for a clinician. It is front line COMMISSIONING and clearly increases value. A continues to remind me of her contribution and often will joke about being the lead commissioner!!

So, the NHS, like all public sectors, is now beginning to express itself with a new word. Perhaps this is a bold claim, but 'value' will be a key term for the next 20 years or so, defining the relationship between outcome and cost of resources used. Porter's (2006) definition of value is set out below.

"Value in any field must be defined around the customer, not the supplier. Value must also be measured by outputs, not inputs. Hence it is patient health results that matter, not the volume of services delivered. But results are achieved at some cost. Therefore, the proper objective is the value of health care delivery, or the patient health outcomes relative to the total cost (inputs) of attaining those outcomes. Efficiency, then, is subsumed in the concept of value. So are other objectives like safety, which is one aspect of outcomes."

Outcomes and Costs

Value then is a key concept and will become even more central to all aspects of service commissioning and provision. Clinicians will know all about value at the level of the individual consultation or episode of care. The outcome of a consultation or a treatment can be defined from a clinical perspective by change in a symptom or risk factor, for example. But we now know that we also have to define outcome in terms of patient experience.

Domain 1	Preventing people from dying prematurely	
Domain 2	Enhancing quality of life for people with long term conditions	Effectiveness
Domain 3	Helping people to recover from episodes of ill health or following injury	
Domain 4	Ensuring that people have a positive experience of care	Patient experience
Domain 5	Treating and caring for people in a safe environment and protecting them from avoidable harm	Safety

FIGURE 3: THE NHS OUTCOMES FRAMEWORK (DOH 2011/2012)

When working at the most important level of the NHS (namely, in clinical practice), the equal cost to both patients and clinicians is **time**. Increasingly, people who manage healthcare are recognised as being clinicians, thousands and thousands of them, even though they do not hold a job called 'commissioner', 'manager' or 'clinical director'. Obviously every clinician manages their own time. Many manage teams and the direction of development for the service. All manage the resources allocated to and within their service, through their actions and all have a duty to maximise value through the elimination of waste and reduction of duplication.

In this position, clinicians determine how the resources will be used efficiently, to get the best outcome at the lowest cost. This concept may be new and perhaps uncomfortable to a few clinicians, particularly as they face ever increasing demands on their service as they draw on their expertise and knowledge. But the issue is to ask how do you decide where to allocate your expertise and knowledge and how do you measure your contribution to the patient experience?

Referring back to the 10 questions above ask:

- What are the right things? How do they improve the outcome and increase value?

But what is value? Whose values do we operate to and do we understand or even consider our patient's values? Are they the same as those of the clinician; are the clinician's values the same as those of the organisation or system they function in? Value means different things to different people; values are like finger prints; because everybody has a different standpoint, clarity is important. But as Porter (2010) reminded us, this is what matters to patients and unites the system.

Value, therefore, is not to be confused with cost cutting or making marginal savings within a departmental budget, but is the clinical benefit achieved for the resource used. This definition is relatively new in dealing with the challenges faced in today's NHS and focuses on two dimensions – quality improvement and cost containment. The requirement of the NHS to maximise the benefit from finite resources means that the choice of service options need to take into account long term sustainability, as well as shorter term financial issues.

The NHS has seen unprecedented funding growth over the past 10 years and latterly, significant levels of increase in spending.

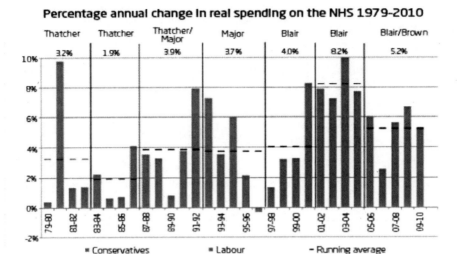

Percentage annual change in real spending on the NHS 1979-2010

Source: The King's Fund (2009). *How cold will it be? Prospects for NHS funding 2011–2017*
© The King's Fund 2010

FIGURE 4: NHS SPENDING 1979-2010

The commissioner needs to remember that the health system as a whole has to be the 'common denominator' for assessing 'equitable' value, built up from the many micro-systems within it. The NHS cannot sustain a perfect value service but there are some minimum standards to improve upon.

So, on the one hand providers of NHS services might claim that value is based on the culture of the organisation or the outcomes which clinicians achieve; on the other, the patient may describe value as their experience or the way they are treated and whether they are treated with dignity and courtesy. It is important to remember that the two are inter-related and both must be considered as equal when increasing value within the NHS. These are critical issues to be considered when introducing value as a concept for change and require careful analysis, for example when confronted with the introduction of a new service or new technology.

Given the demographics and ageing population, need and demand will continue to grow faster than the funds and resources available. This historical upward trend in the use of NHS resources is driven by inexorable demand, which is frequently supported by clinicians and healthcare organisations whose own imperatives are to expand and provide more services. Sometimes new interventions are introduced without a sound evidence base, too often without ceasing other ways of working or paying attention to the impact on the health system as a whole. This can lead to both duplication and fragmentation of services and reduce value.

This conundrum is frequently fuelled by the emergence of new drugs or medical technologies. We, the public and clinicians are often keen to embrace such innovations and introduce them into a clinical setting, even though we do not always understand the implications. Will they bring benefit to our patients or the wider population? May they yield only a marginal enhancement of outcome or benefit just a small number of patients? The question posed by Rowe (2006) is that when resources are finite and that large funding increases are no longer viable, compounded by health costs outstripping overall economic growth, might the NHS need to implement value based purchasing and create a "learning health system"; where, data sharing and transparency can enable patients and the public to have a better understand of health conditions, coupled with a need to manage complex care systems better to increase value. There is also the issue of the extent to which such practices can push clinicians to change behaviour? Could we see perhaps a change with investment going into those programmes where there are known good outcomes, say to reduce obesity and subsequent morbidly from the increased risk of diabetes, rather than investing in new technology, of which the outcomes and gains are unknown?

This highlights a particular issue for consideration and it is this: where to invest finite resources to maximise value. Too frequently resource allocation is made in isolation of a system-wide clinical process on how or where resources could be deployed along a pathway of care to gain greater value. This can be illustrated by the patient with knee pain, referred by the GP to the orthopaedic clinic. Is the referral for advice, physiotherapy, treatment or surgical intervention? There is no doubt that some patients do not experience the anticipated benefit from a surgical intervention. There are others whose expectations are achieved, but there is too often little debate about, say, the wider pathway and how to allocate resources between improving the quality of care and achieving benefit for all patients within existing systems.

Doing things better, safer, cheaper – is necessary but not sufficient.

Value can be measured by improving quality and safety, because the outcome of care is then enhanced.

Value = good outcomes plus cost minus bad outcomes

Value can, therefore, be defined by the relationship between outcome and cost. Providing a service at a lower cost increases value, as long as reducing that cost does not affect the outcome. The cost of care previously has been expressed primarily in terms of money – although for clinicians, their time, skills, knowledge and experience are often as important a constraint as money. Patient time, however, is too often left out of consideration – they are called 'patients' after all! But to reflect, do we have the right clinician seeing the right patient at the right time?

COACH B

B had a senior role within a management team; although a manager by title, he always described himself as a senior manager with a clinical background. B was introduced to me by his Chief Executive, when he was seeking some support and advice on how to make changes to help his clinical team become more efficient. B had used his knowledge and experience very well in describing the benefits to patients and to fellow clinicians, of what he proposed and the reasons for it – as well as the benefits it would bring. The blockage to making this happen though had surprised and disappointed B, to a point where he was considering moving on to seek alternative employment.

We explored how B was perceived by his clinical and management colleagues and in particular, what he thought his unique contribution was to the team. B revealed that he had used his clinical appreciation of the need for change and was working on the "hearts and minds " of his colleagues, but did acknowledge he spent most of his time working with his clinical colleagues – where he felt safer and more comfortable; he had not connected very well with his management team.

Working with B was fun and encouraging as he soon realised that the barrier was a situation he had allowed to happen, but could easily remedy it as he pointed out; it was a case of a difference of language not principle!

B spent time adopting his allies beyond the clinical family and identified who he could work with to get the changes in place; after all as he kept reminding me, they are going to benefit patients! He also learned to stand aside and guide, letting others manage the change whilst he worked where he was comfortable - with his clinical team.

B did complete the change programme and introduced new ways of working and has become more respected as a clinical leader, which is comforting to B who claims he never wanted to be a just a manager.

Doing this better, safer, cheaper is absolutely essential but not sufficient. It is also essential to do the right things. Doing the wrong things better, safer, cheaper is not the strategy for the 21st century.

Ask yourself:

- Do my patients have a shared understanding of the interventions and potential benefits/harm?
- Do my colleagues have a shared understanding of the evidence?
- Do my colleagues have a shared understanding of the higher and lower value activities?
- Are there any changes I would make to increase the value from our service?

Doing the right things

The right things are those of high value; lower value things can be described as activities which:

- have clear evidence that they are ineffective or do more harm than good;
- have no evidence of effectiveness, but are not being delivered in a context that would allow evidence to be gathered to judge effectiveness;
- have evidence of effectiveness, but are being offered to patients whose characteristics are different from those in the research;
- use resources which would produce more value (a better balance of benefit to harm), if invested in some other service for the same group of patients.

To derive optimal maximum value from NHS resources, those resources must be allocated to different geographical populations or different patient groups optimally; but for every person who utilises resources, most of whom are clinicians, the principal causes of lower value healthcare are:

- patients choosing interventions without all the facts, particularly about the probability of benefit **and** the probability of harm;

- clinicians choosing to:
  - □ introduce new interventions or increase the intensity of interventions without switching resources from interventions of lower value;
  - □ continue with longstanding practices for which there is no evidence of value;
- unknown variation in policy and practice, much of which is unwarranted by variation in the incidence or prevalence of disease.

This is shown in the diagram below where the vertical is the amount of benefit and the horizontal is the volume of service, or resource invested and we can see that as we put in more and more resource, benefit increases and then flattens off. This is known as the law of diminishing return. There is also unfortunately the risk of harms increasing, for as we invest more, we may treat people at greater risk of harm or reduced benefits. There comes a point, according to Donabedian (2003) – known as the point of optimality - when you invest further resource, the value drops off.

When optimality is achieved, value is at a maximum. Commissioners need to balance this challenge when investing finite resources, remembering that allocating more money does not always add equal benefit or improved outcome, but to ensure that the patient and the wider population benefits equally and that resources increase value and improve outcomes.

The optimal relationship between resources, benefit and harm (Gray 2011) offers a fresh way to look at investment and ask where and when to invest to gain greatest benefit and better outcomes, Clinicians and patient groups often desire maximally effective healthcare, but for those who pay for healthcare, in a time in which need and demand are greater than the resources that are available, optimality is a more appropriate objective. When optimality is achieved, value is at a maximum. (Gray 2011)"

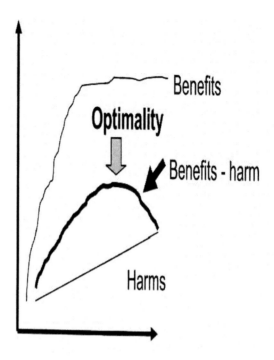

FIGURE 5: OPTIMALITY CURVE
With permission (Gray 2011)

There is a fundamental issue to consider here, that is that not all service improvements require more or additional funding. There is much to be gained by reviewing the current service and refreshing the way it is provided, thus releasing resource from one part of the system to promote more value elsewhere. To some, the concept that the system can "over resource/over-provide" without gaining an equal amount of return is sometimes puzzling. However, the priority must be to ensure resources are being directed to those areas of highest value, thus improving quality, increasing value and getting better outcomes and this will become ever more important.

There is the need, of course, to strike the right balance by constantly evaluating whether investments are gaining the level of benefits expected for the patient and the system. Clinicians are ideally placed to understand this and to have that conversation with their patients and wider population. Managers are ideally placed to recognise when resources could be redirected to other parts of a system to gain more value. The challenge is bringing these parties together, with the patient experience as the catalyst to promote change, to understand and agree when sufficient resource has been allocated and to be brave to make changes necessary.

3

PATIENTS AND POPULATION PLANNING

I t is absolutely right that the patient alongside you is the most important patient at that point in time. The question is, do you assess only the needs of that individual or the population beyond that consultation? Well, it has to be both if we are not to create a system which remains reactive to demand with a dependency on hospitals and buildings. We need to take the information and learning from each and every patient to help us shape services for the wider population.

In preparing care plans with the patient, we need to make a conscious shift away from the large scale institutional based commissioning, which seeks efficiency gains from organisations or reductions in activity. Instead, we should focus on planning integrated care around systems which make a difference to the patients, the population and the clinician as well as maximise value.

Planning

The word "planning" is described as the complex of interrelated decisions about the allocation of available resources.

Planning has four essential properties.

1. Planning is anticipatory decision making.
2. Planning involves a system of decisions.
3. Planning takes place in a dynamic context.

The **Fourth** and last characteristic of planning derives from the third: **the consequences of doing nothing to the system being planned for are more likely than not to be "undesirable."**

Much of the debate about commissioning to date has focused on the margins, making small scale change with "new monies" or released savings. This is unlikely to be sustainable, although it matters. It is even more important to focus on the main budget – not simply on the margin, but on the whole investment that has been made already, as Dr Peter Brambleby emphasises in the Croydon health report 2010. For example, an intense debate with clinicians over £300,000 for some new development, when those same clinicians are currently spending £100 million on a particular programme, is focusing on the wrong issue. The same can be claimed about involving in a debate about investments in programmes such as "urgent care", which is likely to be very different for somebody with a mental health problem and different again for another individual with a respiratory failure. They may both be in need of urgent care but should we be planning for the same system to respond to the very different needs just because it is urgent? We need to start thinking through programmes of care, a whole pathway, self-care, through managed care to include urgent needs, not continue to plan on the basis that whatever the condition presented, the NHS can perform the same organisational miracles to meet their needs just because it is termed as urgent!.

To focus on the programme itself, for example, musculoskeletal disease, clinicians, patients, public health and agencies external to the NHS all need to be engaged with the musculoskeletal community, generalists and specialists to ask them to describe what is the best value for the patients? What plans and systems need to be developed to improve outcomes now and over the next three years? They need to identify who leads which part of the pathway. They also need to spell out the implications and consequences of their investment decisions on the whole pathway, not only on the visibly high activity and intervention parts, important that they are.

Programme budgeting for better value decision-making

This particular disease-based approach, not surprisingly, reflects the way in which medical knowledge is organised through the Medical Subject Headings of the National Library of Medicine. It also reflects the pattern of specialisation within health services in almost every country in the world.

Programme budgeting was developed by the US Department of Defence and clearly described by Enthoven (2005) in the excellent read, **"How much is Enough?"**. He observed that:

> 'the fundamental idea behind Planning-Programming Budgeting System (PPBS) was decision making based on explicit criteria of the national interest in defense programs, as opposed to decision making by compromise among various institutional, parochial, or other vested interests.' (3)

There are six 'basic' ideas:

- 'decision making based on explicit criteria in the national interest;
- the consideration of the needs and costs together;
- the explicit consideration of alternatives at the top level;
- active use of analytic staff at the policy making top level; by an alternative, we mean a balanced, feasible solution to the problem, not a straw man chosen to make a course of action preferred by the originating staff look better by comparison;
- a plan ... which projected into the future the foreseeable implications of current decisions;
- each analysis should be made open to all interested parties.'

A programme is a set of systems with a common knowledge base and a common budget.

The focus of the programme may be on either a group of health problems or a population. The International Classification of Diseases classifies health problems as set out in the table below.

Programme budgeting data has been collected annually within the NHS, from PCT submissions since 2003/04. Data are collected for the 23 main programmes of care (below) based on the World Health Organisations international Classification of Diseases (ICD10).

Table 2: ICD Classification

Infectious diseases	
Cancers and tumours	
Disorders of blood	
Endocrine, nutritional and metabolic	
Mental health disorders	
Problems of learning disability	
Neurological	
Problems of vision	
Problems of hearing	
Problems of circulation	
Problems of the respiratory system	
Dental problems	
Problems of gastrointestinal system	
Problems of skin	
Problems of musculoskeletal system	
Problems due to trauma and injuries	
Problems of genito-urinary system	
Maternity and reproductive health	
Conditions of neonates	
Adverse effects and poisoning	
Healthy individuals	
Social care needs	
Other	

The table above identifies the list of the 23 categories. Ask yourself if you can place the top three in order of spend based on 2008/9 submissions for the nation, and then identify how many millions you believe are spent in each category? Now, ask yourself whether there were £200m, £400m, £800m or more allocated to the highest spend category. Finally, knowing your population where would you allocate the resources?

Now refer to the next table to see how much resource is allocated by each category

Table 3: Allocations made for Programme Budgets 2008-2009

Estimated England level gross expenditure by programme budget		2008/9 – £000s
1	Infectious diseases	1,410.980m
2	Cancers and tumours	5,134,948m
3	Disorders of blood	1,253,786m
4	Endocrine, nutritional and metabolic	2,526,152m
5	Mental health disorders	10,425,840m
6	Problems of learning disability	2,916,182m
7	Neurological	3,683,873m
8	Problems of vision	1,664,102m
9	Problems of hearing	417,167m
10	Problems of circulation	7,420,201m
11	Problems of the respiratory system	4,247,325m
12	Dental problems	3,087,416m
13	Problems of gastrointestinal system	4,097,920m
14	Problems of skin	1,794,226m
15	Problems of musculoskeletal system	4,212,469m
16	Problems due to trauma and injuries	3,299,792m
17	Problems of genito-urinary system	4,000,641m
18	Maternity and reproductive health	3,100,821m
19	Conditions of neonates	1,101,470m
20	Adverse effects and poisoning	955,442m
21	Healthy individuals	1,908,832m
22	Social care needs	3,156,039m
23	Other	24,836,323m
Total gross expenditure		96,814,987m

It is important to acknowledge that the approach to programme budgeting, based on healthcare conditions and ICD codes, has a number of limitations. It is difficult to classify spend before diagnosis is made and increasingly many people have more than one condition. This needs to be borne in mind, but does not justify the popular claim that programme budgeting cannot be used to help clinician's and commissioners alike to allocate resources to improve outcomes. On the contrary, we need to continue to use, improve and refine programme budgeting and find a way to handle the data combining a disease-based approach to programming with a population-based approach. For example one programme being focused on people with four or more conditions which could be called a 'frail elderly' programme – or a programme for people with complex chronic needs. Similarly, a programme for single people who are homeless is one that focuses on a population of people who share a common characteristic.

The principle underlying programme budgeting is very simple. It offers a method of understanding spend and how or where resources are allocated and what benefits they bring to a population. The method then allows clinicians to engage in the debate about where those resources are best applied and more so, what priorities should be set for a known population and which data should be recorded and used to measure outcomes.

Between programme - marginal analysis

Having decided first how to allocate resources to different geographical populations, and appreciating the use of those resources within a disease group, the questions that need to be tackled by people who pay for or manage healthcare resources are set out below.

- Has money been distributed to different patient groups, e.g. people with cancer and people with lung disease, in such a way as to maximise value?
- Are all the interventions being offered likely to confer a good balance of benefit and harm, at affordable cost, for this group of patients?
- Are the patients most likely to benefit from, and least likely to be harmed by, the intervention clearly defined?
- Could each patient's experience be improved?
- How is effectiveness being maximised?
- Are the risks of care being minimised?
- Can costs be reduced without increasing harm or reducing benefit?

The first question in this list focuses on the allocation of resources – the analysis of the effect of moving them between two different groups of patients (for example by asking: 'should we switch some resources from mental health to respiratory disease or vice versa?'). This is called marginal analysis and seeks to produce greater benefit from shifting resources toward greater identified need.

To maximise value this type of approach has to be taken and the common currency used must not only be financial but also QALYs (Quality Adjusted life Years) or DALYs (Disability Adjusted Life Years). This is, however, difficult to manage at a local level. The aim, as described earlier, is to reach the point of optimality, or maximum allocative efficiency.

Furthermore, the use of programme budgeting has another advantage; i.e. allowing localities to compare themselves against similar areas. This simple approach is to see how the relationship between spend and outcome for one population compares with spend and outcome for another. The information allowing this comparison is now provided by the Department of Health, the Information Centre, and the Public Health Observatories. Very simply, spend is related to outcome, and each Primary Care Trust can compare their spend and outcome not only with that of all other Primary Care Trusts but also with Primary Care Trusts looking after similar populations. These tools are highlighted in the next chapter.

4

DEVELOPING BEST VALUE SYSTEMS, NETWORKS AND PATHWAYS

D isease and ill-health respects no geographical or organisational boundary. Yet as previously demonstrated, we often hear of a great deal of NHS time spent discussing the shape of bureaucracies and organisations. Clinical Commissioning Groups may be in danger of going the same way, with more of a focus on the numbers of GP practices and the geography, rather than an understanding of the population's health needs and building a system locally to address those needs.

With the constant scrutiny from the media and some public focus remaining on buildings and structures (frequently referred to as 'hospitals' or 'centres' as being representative of the NHS), it is of little surprise that discussions relating to health and well-being are largely restricted to NHS buildings – with a sharper focus on secondary and specialist services. This is not the full picture of the NHS, since these hospital-based organisations only deal with a minority of care, critical and important though that is. The majority of care and NHS services are provided outside the hospital, in general medical practices, community pharmacists and by other generalist clinicians working outside of hospitals.

For some unidentifiable reason, the hidden work of general medical practice and other community-based generalist services, community nurses, physiotherapists, dieticians and many more does not gain as much media and political attention. Therefore, it is not surprising that the public maintains a myopic and historical view of the NHS, with a focus on bricks and mortar rather than systems of care. It is important to remember though that the system of care, or the way the NHS collectively provides care for the public, is the driver, not a structure, for value and quality. We need to put more focus on the system we function in and imagine how good they can be if clinician's pull together and managers support change.

Systems

What is meant by a system though? Is it easy to describe the system of care we work in? It is all too easy to believe and claim that we work in a system covering a broad network with one managerial process functioning at all levels, with the patient or patients at the heart of the system, and the organisation built around that. But do we really have this?

It is perhaps more of a concept than a reality, as it is difficult for many clinicians to describe their "system" to colleagues or our public – in particular, the part they play within that system in both their clinical or managerial role, and more importantly how it benefits the patients. More frequently than not it is described as fragmented not integrated.

Let us explore this a little more. How often do we accept *the system* as it appears, described more as a bureaucracy, and how frequently do we review the system and ask ourselves if it is truly adding the value we desire and which patients deserve?

COACH C

C operates as a senior manager working in a "network" covering a large geographical area, over many organisational boundaries. She had asked for support to resolve the challenges she was facing with having too many managers and not sufficient time to deliver what they wanted.

C defined the real issue as being the complex arrangements she faced for line management and her own performance reporting. She rarely felt comfortable when discussing her role with her managers. A contributing factor we identified was the previous upheaval and reorganisation of the PCTs, to which she worked, thus changing her reporting structure. C would say that she no longer knew who to report to or how to keep her managers informed and C often spoke about having too many people telling her what to do, that she had to report across the system; beyond her own tier which was causing her distress. The complex accountability was preventing C performing at the optimal level and we explored the lines of accountability and paid attention to her line management and the recent changes in her reporting.

The issue we worked with was the accountability and the responsibility C held within the network and within the new structures. It became clear to C that she in reality avoided seeking clarity as it was difficult to share the added value of the network to the new infrastructure.

C created opportunities to describe how the network could add value, in the new management arena, and identified that there were other resources and teams that she would have to work with. C chose not to do this, deciding to move on to seek a different role, away from the network.

According to Ackoff (1993), calling a group of healthcare organisations a 'system' has become common practice. As he and others have noted, however, true systems involve a functionally related group of interacting, inter-related or interdependent elements forming a complex whole with a common aim. In simpler terms, system elements must be capable of working together to achieve shared goals; otherwise they are merely individual parts with separate missions.

So, taking a system as described and supported by Dennis (2007) who claims that a system *'is an integrated series of parts with a clearly defined goal'*, ask yourselves what system you work in, what are the parts, and what contributions you make to achieve a single goal and how consensus is reached on agreeing that goal. What do you contribute to the system and what influence can you have on making sure the system is well designed and delivers optimal care for the patient?

Using a pie chart as a framework, describe your system to show how much of your time goes into each of the 4 segments labelled as:

> A: The system
> B: Links with others
> C: Your Role
> D: Your Key Objectives

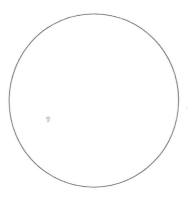

FIGURE 6: YOUR PIE CHART OF TIME UTILIZATION

How do we work in a system and do we all know our impact?

COACH D

D is a seasoned and experienced GP who sought my help with making an impact outside the clinical and small geographical arena in which he was comfortable. He wanted to be recognised as a leader by his colleagues and to be in a position of influence within the local health care environment.

D had recently undertaken the lead in some local work, which he had enjoyed and decided that " time had come" for him to do something different and to be a leader, changing the way services were planned and delivered around the locality in which he worked.

D would say that *"existing practice can be quite comfortable, so you do need the right circumstances to make a change"*. He acknowledged that it was quite a large gamble, but it was the right time to try. We spent some time working out what D perceived to be the blocks in the system, preventing him from being seen as a leader and identifying that what was actually stopping him was his own approach - he wanted to be a leader and seen as a change agent and deliver it – all in one go!

D worked a lot on his own image and behaviour, identifying that he wanted to change things but recognised that he needed a process and support from others to help him do it. He also acknowledged he was doing this from the heart, with hope that others would follow –because as he often said, "it makes sense!"

The work D focused on was to put together a narrative and to share his story with colleagues, encouraging them to understand what and why he believed it was important to change. The biggest change D made, however, was to create the right engagement to encourage others to see that they could contribute. His enthusiasm and encouragement proved a great success to a growing band of clinicians promoting better care for their patients.

On final reflection D appreciated that leadership comes in different forms and that being a leader does not require you to do it all. Helping to bring about a change in other people's behaviour was his success.

Some of the insight reveals that there can be a tendency for front-line clinicians to adopt a blame culture when looking at their own clinical practice, claiming that the management and their bureaucracy will not let them do the right things for their patients. Sadly, this is often a claim made in isolation of the reality and the word 'bureaucracy' has become demonised. Perrow (1970) claimed that

> 'Bureaucracy' is a dirty word, both to the average person and to many specialists on organizations. It suggests rigid rules and regulations, a hierarchy of offices, narrow specialization of personnel, an abundance of offices or units which can hamstring those who want to get things done, impersonality, resistance to change. Yet every organization of any significant size is bureaucratized to some degree or, to put it differently, exhibits more or less stable patterns of behaviour based upon a structure of roles and specialized tasks. Bureaucracy, in this sense, is another word for structure.'

It is important that clinicians appreciate this and reflect as to how it impacts on their behaviour and how it impacts on the system in which they work. Only then can they understand how to use the bureaucracy to help them achieve the delivery of that single goal of improving patient care, within the system in which they function.

One of the most striking behaviours during periods of significant change is to blame the organisation for deflecting clinicians from providing the care they want to give to their patients and population. This is experienced by many to some degree. There are examples where the executive team and senior managers are either not communicating the shared narrative of change, in particular the benefits to patients and populations. The integration of front-line clinicians and patients, either directly or indirectly through patient representative groups, can be a way to overcome this separation of planning, avoiding the 'top-down' feeling many clinicians grumble about during a period of change.

The system of care is of primary importance; and so is the bureaucracy within it, but one should not spend too much time trying to oppose the organisation of the bureaucracy. Rather, clinicians should help shape it and be involved. The real challenge is to remember and focus on what contribution clinicians can make to patient care and to the service with their skills and experience, and how together they can make the system of care work to improve health outcomes.

During stressful periods of change, it is important to acknowledge that, as a clinician maintaining a focus on clinical care, it can sometimes feel that your contribution can be dismissed or forgotten. This is unsettling. It is critical that you review your impact and remind yourself and others of the important contribution you are making to the system, demonstrating the significant part your skills contribute to that collective goal.

This can be particularly difficult and challenging; particularly when it is often without good leadership and support,. The reality is that front-line clinicians often feel disempowered during times of significant change. This can lead to different behaviours and inertia, or disorganisation rather than organisation, with many clinicians adopting a perception that it is 'them and us', which is considered later.

This needs to be addressed with urgency to avoid stagnation and drift. It is imperative that clinicians work with managers and leaders to describe and communicate the changes in a narrative and language that can be used and understood by patients.

COACH E

E was seeking some help with her career during a period of significant change, moving out of a long established clinical/management role into a full time management position, with no patient contact. This was her first step away from direct patient care, a senior nurse well respected and a natural clinical leader, able to communicate effectively and confidently with colleagues, patients and relatives.

E had held several roles with the title clinical manager and had comfortably stepped into management roles on occasions, albeit on each occasion for short periods of time before reverting back to full-time clinical roles. They were as E put it "task and finish groups", but on each occasion E could see the line of sight to patients, retaining a case load.

E had clearly reflected on the issues of moving into a management role and what it meant to her working without direct patient contact, identifying that her biggest challenge was to maintain credibility with colleagues.

On this occasion we focussed on her strengths and how she was perceived by colleagues, in particular, how much of that was her retaining a case-load and how much was due to her skills, experience and knowledge which she brought to the system.

This revealed another issue. During times that E had stepped up into other roles she had observed the challenging relationships with her peers and managers and the negative impact this often had as a "them and us" culture prevailed.

E did leave clinical practice and move into a management role and is a very successful senior manager, considering a future in a Board level role. She worked through her anxieties and concerns of not being taken seriously as a manager, but informed me recently that her own appreciation of her strengths, the understanding of what she contributes and her confidence to constantly challenge the "them and us" culture has made the move more testing but more rewarding.

Another important behaviour to avoid during periods of significant change is adopting a critical commentator's role without offering solutions and improvements. It is essential that we do not all become observers and commentators. It is crucial that the focus remains on the patients; they rely on us, our professionalism and our advocacy. There is a need to understand the changes and the impact they will have on us as individuals and on our role, and the parts of the service in which we function. It is a clinician's duty to articulate and describe the service in terms that the patients and public understand, alleviate fear and distress, and articulate what good care looks like. Furthermore, patients rarely want to try and understand the full details of any NHS management or structural change going on around them. What they do want to know is that they can access the system and will receive timely, safe and effective care, reflecting their values. The duty on clinicians is to remember the patient and this is our key role during these periods of change.

Building the system: A practical way forward

Every system needs a single high-level aim with which all professionals and patients can identify and readily acknowledge as being the collective purpose. Without this there is conflict and drift. The aim requires a clear narrative, telling the "story" of the "what and the why". That aim then has to be complemented by a set of objectives through which all those involved, patients and professionals, can focus their activities, measure and evaluate progress.

Setting objectives

Objectives are needed in every area where performance and results matter and where they affect the sustainability and enhancement of networks and systems. The narrative should describe clearly the objectives and measurements in a way that enables us to do five things:

1. to organize and explain the whole programme;
2. to test these statements in actual experience;
3. to plan or predict behaviour;
4. to appraise the soundness of decisions when they are still being made; and
5. to enable practising clinicians to analyse their own experience and, as a result, improve their performance.

So, each system has to have a set of objectives. As an example, a draft set of objectives for an epilepsy programme, developed in a RightCare (www.rightcare.nhs.uk) workshop for a population based service, is set out below. The workshop was attended by a mixture of patients, public and professionals, all with an interest in making the programme of care for epilepsy more cohesive and integrated. The workshop concluded with the following objectives, designed to help their system achieve its high-level aim of *'helping people with epilepsy live fulfilling lives'*.

1. to organize and explain the whole programme;
2. to test these statements in actual experience;
3. to plan or predict behaviour;
4. to appraise the soundness of decisions when they are still being made; and
5. to enable practising clinicians to analyse their own experience and, as a result, improve their performance.

- To diagnose epilepsy quickly and accurately.
- To treat effectively and with minimal side effects.
- To help the child and their family to adjust to the diagnosis and to minimise handicap.
- To involve children and their families, both individually and collectively, in disease management.
- To promote research.
- To develop all the professionals and practitioners involved in epilepsy care.
- To make the best use of resources.
- To produce an Annual Report for the population served.

The objectives are of two types. There are those which relate to clinical issues which are analogues of the traditional clinical activity (to diagnose accurately and quickly, for example), and those which relate to the use of resources for a population. The latter though are often overlooked by clinicians when they are first involved in objective setting.

Practical steps

Objective setting is usually relatively easy. Here is one way to approach it – using Tweetshire as the area, with a population of 1.5 million:

- Gather the community of practice – all the key organisations and individuals, including

patient and carer representatives; don't worry about numbers, this can be done with a big group.
- Inform them that the task is to agree the objectives of the service and show them a table with objectives, criteria, standards and outcomes, such as that shown below.

Table 4: System Planning

Objectives	Criteria	Outcomes	Standards

- Put up a draft aim, the high level statement, for example: *'The aim of the epilepsy service for Tweetshire is to minimise the impact of epilepsy on the life of the person who has it.'*
- Ask the group to discuss this aim in twos and threes and take feedback; redraft, concentrating on the important words like 'impact' or 'minimise'.
- Explain that this may be revisited after the next step which is to set the objectives.
- Give them an example of an objective such as *'to treat effectively and with minimal side effects';* tell the group they cannot use this one but they might want to modify it and that each objective needs to start with the word 'to'. Then give them five minutes or so, in their twos or threes, and take feedback.
- Write up objectives as they appear and then show a set of objectives like that given earlier in this section; usually people are good at identifying the type of objectives that reflect clinical practice; objectives relating to diagnosis and treatment, and are weak at identifying more managerial types of objectives, such as 'to make the best use of resources'.

Close the meeting and agree that a draft set of objectives will be written up and circulated for comment, and then move on to the next step - identify criteria.

Choosing criteria

For each objective there needs to be one or more criteria to allow progress towards the objective – or lack of it – to be measured, this is critical, without a measure there is no progress.

The choice of criteria is perhaps the more challenging aspect of this process as it needs to balance two variables – validity and feasibility. In general the more valid the criterion, the more expensive and less feasible it is to collect. The choice of criteria may also be influenced by the selection of data that are currently being collected. But the choice should not be restricted to those data; it requires improvement. Priority should then be given to agreeing objectives and identifying valid, feasible criteria – making the best use of currently collected data, not waiting for the 100% consolidation of data sources.

However, it is important not to be constrained by the current dataset because it may relate to objectives set, (or data arbitrarily chosen) in preceding years, and not to the current set of objectives for the system. It is worth a mention here that one issue frequently identified is the use, or lack of useable data and the quest by many to seek the gold-standard data source which is rarely available. There is a need to agree the source, analysis and application of data and make progress – it is necessary to continually refine and improve the data but it is not good enough to avoid action whilst a few keep fine tuning data!

Fortunately, it is usually possible to reconcile these issues, and with the maxim "Do Once Locally and Share', groups of clinicians and patients can work with information specialists to identify the datasets that were needed for many common conditions.

Practical steps

For each objective, one or more criteria need to be identified. This takes a little time and the input of two critical contributions. It is essential to include people who think about measurement, and people who do research.

It usually needs a separate session from the workshop for objective-setting, in part because of time. This is because it is often helpful to have clinical or health service researchers there, even if they know little about the condition being discussed. Identifying the criteria that measure quickness and accuracy of diagnosis to assess the outcomes related to this objective is analogous to designing a research protocol.

- Take one objective at a time.
- Tell participants not to worry about whether or not the information they wanted was being collected.
- Give them five minutes to work in pairs or threes.
- Take feedback from the pair on the left and write it up exactly.
- Ask if any other pair had anything radically different; if so, take that too; if not, ask participants to crawl over the proposed criterion.
- Reach agreement on the criterion, then go back to the objective and remind people that the meaning of terms is often clarified by discussions about data.
- Reach agreement that the objective does or does not need changing in light of this discussion.
- Close the debate on this criterion; do not try to define the data terms that will be required to produce the criterion – that involves different types of people, e.g. information technology experts.
- Move on to the next objective.

Measuring outcome

Outcomes are an elusive concept - Measurement is not, but is frequently vague in description within most programmes. Everyone talks about 'outcomes' with different meanings and Donabedian's work, published in 1966, distinguished structure, process and outcome can expressed his meanings in the following way.

The structure of care – based on robust evidence: how should treatment and care be structured in order to maximise the chance of a good outcome for the patient?

The processes of care – based on robust evidence: what are the things that should be done to maximise the chance of a good outcome for the patient?

The outcomes of care – what actually happens to the health of the patient, the outcome, as a result of the treatment and care they receive?

From Donabedian (1966) article 'Evaluating the Quality of Medical Care'.

This definition has stood the test of time but there have been developments in its use. One has been the distinction between primary and secondary outcomes, with the primary outcome the real objective of treatment, as demonstrated by Hickson *et al.* in 2007:

> 'Primary outcome: occurrence of antibiotic-associated diarrhoea.
> Secondary outcome: presence of C.difficile toxin in the diarrhoea.'

In addition, there has been increasing use, and criticism, of intermediate outcomes. In a cardiovascular disease prevention programme, the primary outcome is obviously measured by the mortality from heart disease, but there are two problems with using this outcome measure.

The first is that it may take many years and a very large population to show this difference. For this reason, intermediate outcomes may be chosen. In this example, this may be about changes in blood lipid levels of the population being studied. The second reason is that the primary outcome may be affected by many factors other than the health service provided, as clearly described by Le Grand (2007).

> 'There is a particular problem with outcomes, in that it is often difficult to attribute a given outcome improvement (such as in the health of a patient) to a particular item of public service (such as a course of medical treatment). For the outcome may in large part be due to a variety of factors that are not within the control of the providers of the service concerned (such as the patient's own recuperative powers). This is one of the reasons why, although both providers and policy makers often pay lip service to the importance of outcomes, in practice they usually give more attention to factors that are more under the control of the service, such as inputs, processes and outputs.'

In chasing outcomes as such, it may become clear that the wording of the objective and the choice of criteria chosen to measure progress may need to be amended. It may seem that there is a straight forward linear process, but the reality is different (Figure 4.2) and it is important that as clinicians you do not constrain your thinking to an expected behaviour, but that you encourage flexibility and try new ways of working.

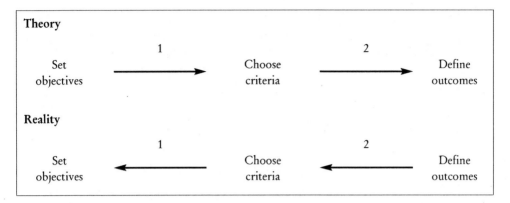

FIGURE 7: THE PROCESS OF REFINING OUTCOMES (GRAY 2011)

Here is an example worked through during a training workshop.

- The aim of the Chronic Obstructive Pulmonary Disease (COPD) Programme is to help people with COPD live a fulfilling life.
- One objective is 'to treat COPD safely and effectively'.
- The network, including patients, tackles the problem.

Table 5: Objective – Outcomes

Objectives	Criteria
To treat patients safely and effectively	- pCO2 measurements of the amount of carbon dioxide in the bloodstream - the patient's reports - feeling better or not - the patient's reports - whether or not they experienced side effects - clinical findings of side effects

- Now, it is essential to distinguish outcomes for the individual patient from outcomes for the system.
- It is only in the last 10 years that the patient's experience of the "humanity of the consultation" *and* their care, became considered an outcome of importance equal to that of clinical effectiveness. However, the example provided shows that the patient's

report is essential to measuring not only their emotional experience but also the clinical effectiveness of their treatment. This has led to the development of PROMs – Patient Reported Outcome Measures - which measure quality from the patient's perspective.

Agreeing quality standards

The work for NICE (The National Institute for Health and Clinical Excellence), is the development of clinical standards. Where these standards are available, they should be used. If they are not yet available, steps need to be taken to agree standards locally until National Institute Clinical Excellence (NICE) has covered the topic. But, remember to document your process, log your decision making and make it transparent, engaging with all parties, including patients and representative groups to agree the standards. Performance and progress can then be measured against the agreed standards. Different levels of standard can be set; for example: a minimum acceptable standard, an achievable standard, or an excellent standard.

The application of these principles in an example for sickle cell disease is shown in the table below.

Table 6: An Example of Programme Standards

Newborn Screening for Sickle Cell Disorders Programme Standards			
Newborn programme objectives	Criteria	Standards	
		Minimum (core)	Achievable (developmental)
Programme outcome Best possible survival for infants detected with a sickle cell disorder by the screening programme	Mortality rates expressed in person years	Mortality rate from sickle cell disease and its complications in children under five of less than four per 1000 person years of life (two deaths per 100 affected children)	Mortality rate in children under five of less than two per 1000 person years of life (one death per 100 children affected)
Programme outcome Accurate detection of all infants born with major clinically significant haemoglobin disorders	Sensitivity of the screening process (offer, test and repeat test)	99% detection for Hb-SS 96% detection for Hb-SC 95% detection for other variants	99.5% for Hb-SS 99% for Hb-SC 97% for other variants

Building networks

A network is a set of individuals and organisations who work together for a common aim. A clear description of networking is provided by Child (2005)

> 'Networking is a broad concept referring to a form of organized transacting that offers an alternative to either markets or hierarchies. It refers to transactions across an organization's boundaries that are recurrent and involve continuing relationships with a set of partners. The transactions are coordinated and controlled on a mutually agreed basis that is likely to require common protocols and systems, but do not necessarily require direct supervision by the organization's own staff.' *(Childs, 2005)*

This example of the meaning of 'networking' is drawn from the RightCare Glossary (www.rightcare.nhs.uk) which will not only provide examples of the meaning of the terms commonly employed, but also emphasise that there is rarely an absolute and final definition of a term. As a consequence, care must be taken to ensure that everyone in a meeting or service is using terms such as 'efficiency' or 'quality' with the same meaning.

One key factor that characterises networks is that they contain a number of organisations. These organisations relate to one another not only through contracts and bureaucratic arrangements – necessary though these sometimes are – but also through trusting relationships.

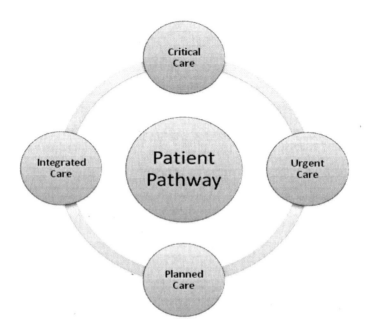

FIGURE 8: INTEGRATED PATIENT PATHWAYS

As suggested earlier, it is important to be clear about the meaning of words and that everybody is working to the same definition and none so more important than the ubiquitous term - Patient Pathway.

Brigato and Jacobs *(2003)* suggest that there are three different things being talked about under the general heading of Integrated Care Pathways and if we agree what they are, then it should make it a lot clearer:

1. The first type of Integrated Care Pathway (ICP) is the actual care process of pathway experienced by each individual patient/client.

2. ICPs are also described as maps that define *best practice* and the *minimum clinical standards* or essential components of care for every patient/client in a given situation. Therefore a care pathway is a standard or universal plan for how a patient/client with a particular condition will be treated.
3. ICPs normally involve physical documentation that is located at the point of care and may replace traditional records.

This documentation is also called the care pathway and is central to the task of patient/client care under the pathway approach, as the care process is clearly presented on the documentation **for all those involved** to see.

Pathways are increasingly used to describe processes and to standardise care, relying on clinicians to deviate from the pathway only when the patient's needs and values require it. NICE is now using pathways as a means of representing its guidance, aware of the fact that many people prefer this style of communication. There is a critical issue to address here though and that is to simply lift national standards and set them to a local environment, undermines the absolute requirement to appreciate the need to contextualise and localise the standards so as to acknowledge the cultural and behavioural issues, which this book has highlighted as a challenge if clinicians are not supported and developed.

So, national pathways do have to be localised to take into account local constraints and opportunities – research projects, for example, but there should be no excuse to either reject them on grounds of "not invented here" or too difficult to implement given local constraints! There are too many examples, across the NHS, of pathways and standards being developed locally but not shared, or worse still, invented and not implemented. These compound the problem faced of duplication and waste, expecting 100 plus organisations to do the same thing and "invent their own" minimises value and we should promote the "do-once-and-share" approach.

The Map of Medicine software is a good example of how the national/local dimensions can function very effectively. (www.mapofmedicine.com) This process, designed to facilitate localisation has evidence based pathways available for local use. The Map of Medicine's system is a model which enables local networks to amend their core pathways to reflect local objectives, whether it be to improve diagnostic rates, explicitly communicate criteria for specific types of care, or identify subgroups of the population that can be seen in a local 'view' of the Map. This localised version then becomes the default version of the Map seen when users in a network log on. An example of a localised Map of Medicine pathway, again for COPD, is shown below (www.mapofmedicine.com)

Local networks, therefore, are able to focus on local requirements rather than having first to understand the evidence base from which a pathway should be derived. This significantly reduces cumulative effort across the country's many networks by avoiding duplicative behaviour. The Map of Medicine also regularly reviews emerging evidence on a monthly basis and, with advice from its clinical advisers, decides when to update its core pathway. These updates are then communicated to local networks which can decide whether and how to change their local objectives and/or pathway. This, again, reduces the effort required across the country to stay abreast of emerging evidence.

Often local networks have already captured their system-specific objectives and tactics, but have struggled to communicate them effectively further afield. The Map of Medicine is able to work with local networks to quickly add their pre-created objectives and tactics into local versions of its pathways, which are then approved by network leaders.

The Map of Medicine has already enabled numerous networks to create local pathways as part of their quality improvement initiatives. There are currently more than 270 localised pathways within the Map.

Although improvements to services can take a significant period of time to show benefit, the Map has enabled local networks to improve the efficacy and safety of services and examples of benefits realised are available on the Map of Medicine (www.mapofmedicine.com).

Deciding how many systems

A system, described earlier, is a set of activities with a common set of objectives, each of which has:

- criteria for measuring progress and expressing the
- outcomes of the system which can be assessed against
- standards of quality, the performance being described in an
- Annual Report.

But how many systems should there be for the population of England? That is a function of many variables, including:

- the incidence and prevalence of condition or conditions;
- the complexity of treatment;

- the need, if any, for heavy capital investment;
- the consequences of diagnostic or treatment failure.

There is probably, for example, a need for fewer epilepsy services than, say, asthma services, based on these criteria. One factor might be the number of specialised neurological services, even though only a small proportion of people are referred to them, because they could report on the referral rates from different paediatric services in their annual report. Those who know how to run services need to use their judgement, based on the evidence such as it is, and their experience.

Clinical commissioning offers a fresh opportunity to review the number and shape of services and how they are organised around the needs of the population. Decisions can then be made to appreciate where the best outcomes can be delivered and what resource is needed to achieve that goal, investing in the right systems and disinvesting in others.

5

INCREASING VALUE BY THE RIGHT INNOVATION AND DISINVESTMENT

I n times of plenty, innovation was funded from new money. In an era when no new money is available, it is still possible for a commissioner to fund an innovation in support of people with chronic obstructive pulmonary disease (COPD), for example, by switching money from the programme budget for cancer or the programme budget for gastrointestinal disease. However, unless there is a compelling case for doing this – expenditure on respiratory disease being in the bottom deciles of spending by the commissioner, for example – the commissioner will expect resources to be found from within the respiratory programme budget.

Within-programme marginal analysis: One Approach

One of the benefits of using programme budgeting is that it relates to specialists and specialties in medicine. As a result, it is possible to compare within any population the amount of resources committed to, for example, asthma, compared with the amount invested in COPD or the management of sleep apnoea, as shown in Figure xx previously on page.

If a decision were made to hold the programme budget constant, then local clinicians and patient groups could be engaged in a debate about the pressures on different services and the priorities that should be given to switching resources from one to another – by analysing the changes at the margin of each of these three system budgets, were they to be increased or decreased.

It is, of course, possible and essential to repeat this type of analysis for any single system within the amount of money committed to COPD. For example, it is possible to consider the benefits and harms of switching resources between smoking cessation to prevent COPD, telephone support for people with COPD, triple therapy, etc.

Intra-system marginal analysis should also challenge the use of resources within each system to maximise value. Thus to continue with the same value before deciding to switch resources from one type of therapy to another, or switching resources between COPD and asthma, it is essential for the question to be asked for each system within the respiratory disease programme budget, 'can more value be derived from the resources within the system?'.

There are two ways of maximising value – i.e. to ensure that:

- the right things are being done, and
- these things are done right.

Doing the right things right is an old management proverb. Quality improvement is primarily concerned with doing things right or, to be more precise, doing things better, safer and cheaper. It is essential to increase value by quality improvement. It is also essential to keep challenging the decisions that have been made to start some activity or to stop some other activity. **Clinicians will, therefore, have to take responsibility for:**

- starting the right things – innovation;
- stopping the right things – disinvestment.

These decisions are not always as tricky as they sound, but are often left out of the debate when trying new techniques or introducing new ways of working. Remember, the work harder or work smarter claim is not enough; clinician's need to accept responsibility for the use of all resources and are in the privileged position to make that a reality.

Taking the example below, based on the Association of Public Health Observatories (APHO www.apho.org.uk) Spend and Outcome tool (SPOT), is a breakdown of a PCT programme budget activity and spends. In the example, programmes are presented by a quadrant along the two axis (spend and outcome) and the commissioners task is to understand this and to review spend against the known needs of the population. They should then ask whether the right investments are being made to gain the best value from resources for that known population.

So, to illustrate, focus on the quadrant in the bottom right hand of the SPOT Ca (cancers). It reveals that spend is high and the outcome poor. But what can commissioners do to address this and allocate resources to the greatest need?

The chart shows the relative spend and outcome for programmes in a PCT, comparing it to similar PCTs in England, as defined by the Office for National Statistics (ONS). There are a range of outcome measures available in the tool for each disease area. Each diamond represents a disease programme and the largest diamonds represent the biggest programmes. The labelling on each quadrant (e.g. higher spend, worse outcome) is there to make the chart easier to read.

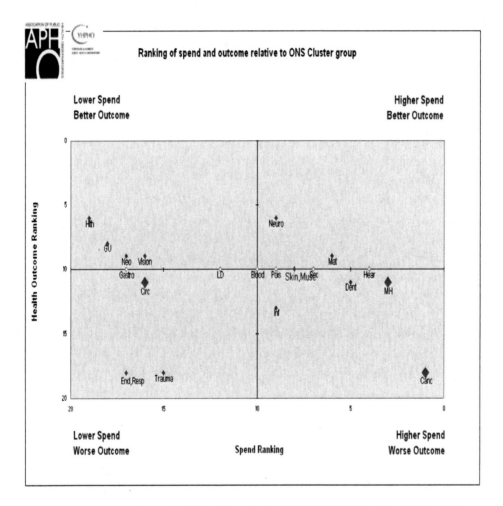

FIGURE 9: TWEETSHIRE PCT SPOT ANALYSIS SHOWING SPEND AND OUTCOMES.

Improving Outcomes: What can clinicians do?

Taking the example above, commissioners need to work with their colleagues to understand the needs and to make some decisions about taking action to improve the desired outcomes through better investments. Clearly, moving resources into one programme budget area will need to reduce in another programme, so being clear about the **aims, outcomes and criteria**, as described above are essential to creating the right system to make the improvements required.

Health Investment – a clinicians' guide and the Challenge

This is a considerable challenge. To be a high spender with poor outcomes is not a desirable place to be. Clinicians do however respond swiftly to this challenge, once it is understood by using knowledge and expertise underpinned by peer review, published and comparative data and clinician led service reviews they, to address this swiftly and efficiently.

The challenge, being a high spender with good outcomes is equally difficult. There are levers in the system, such as best practice tariff, critical evaluation of coding and referral processes and improvement tools (www.institute.nhs.uk) to assist. There are also tools available (www.apho.org.uk) to help identify better investments and to improve health outcomes and increase value. Practically this can be done by a number of steps.

Step 1: Identify relative spend across programmes at CCG level

As a starting point, Clinical commissioners could use the **programme budgeting benchmarking tool** to identify how much is spent by their host PCT on each disease group compared to other similar PCTs. The tool can be used to identify how a PCT's allocation is spent across the 23 diseases and their respective subcategories e.g. lung cancer, breast cancer. The tool also shows the PCT's spend per head compared with PCTs nationally, locally or with similar characteristics.

The **Inpatient Variation Expenditure Tool** (www.networks.nhs.uk) can also be used to look at potential investment opportunities for the higher spending programmes.

Step 2: Identify the relationship between spend and health outcomes at PCT level

Once clinical commissioning groups have an understanding of expenditure across the different disease categories, the next stage is to examine the relationship between spend and a range of health outcomes. The Spend and Outcome Tool (SPOT) enables GP commissioners to identify how the expenditure and outcomes of their PCT compare to others nationally, within similar demographic areas, and against any other individual PCT of interest. This is a good starting point to determine local priorities.

Through this process, clinical commissioners should be able to identify a number of programmes (currently at PCT level but can be broken down into systems or smaller groupings) that may benefit from further investigation. The next step is to examine whether these programmes are also an issue for any the constituent GP Practices.

Step 3: Identify the relative spend and outcomes across programmes at GP commissioner level

With an understanding of which programmes are relatively high, or low spending and which have better, or worse outcomes across the PCT, the next stage is to examine whether these are the same for the constituent practices. To do this, **NHS Comparators** (www.nhscomparators.nhs.uk) can be used to look at relative spend on primary care prescribing, outpatients and inpatients across programmes, offering a more complete reflection of health spend.

To identify corresponding outcomes across the GP commissioner, a number of sources can help. If the GP commissioner's population is large and broadly corresponds to a local authority boundary, the **Health Profiles** published by the Association of Public Health Observatories, provide a range of health outcomes. If this is not the case, the PCT's Joint Strategic Needs Assessment (JSNA) will contain a section showing health outcomes at a smaller geographical scale.

Step 4: Identify the drivers of spend in greater detail

Once programmes have been identified which have potential health investment or disinvestment possibilities, the next step is to identify the drivers of spend. NHS Comparators can be applied to achieve a detailed investigation. This tool can examine a whole range of activities which affect overall spend at practice level e.g. prevalence rates, prescribing rates, outpatient attendances, elective and emergency admissions. To make comparisons fairer, the tool can be used to assess practices with similar needs profiles. Both spend and activity volumes at disease group (programme) level can be compared.

APHO – General Practice Profiles can be used to compare Quality & Outcomes Framework (QOF) measures to examine measurement and management in primary care. At the end of this step, GPs and other commissioners should have a better understanding of relative expenditure, health outcomes and drivers of spend at a fairly detailed level.

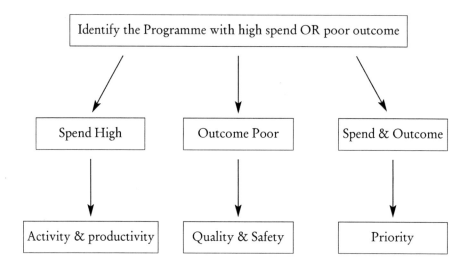

FIGURE 10: MAPPING SPEND AND OUTCOMES

Step 5: Implementation

Once potential programmes have been identified for further investigation, then a reliable method, such as marginal analysis, is helpful to prioritise investments that deliver the greatest health benefits for patients. This stage requires clinical commissioners to analyse, in detail, their spend and outcomes, in light of local knowledge of their population and services. It is essential that a wide range of clinicians are involved in this process.

6

MAXIMISING VALUE FOR THE PATIENT

I n this chapter the book will focus on the issue of maximising value for the patient. How for instance do we know that what we are providing is really providing value for our patient or patients? Moreover, in what ways can we maximize such value?

Variation and Unwarranted variation

There will always be variation in a modern and innovative health service. The process is to identify which variation is acceptable and, more importantly, explicable to the public, clinicians and managers – probably in that order!

It is also important to distinguish here between 'variation' and the often misused and emotive term 'postcode lottery', which has found its way into the healthcare lexicon to describe poor provision or an absence of a service in a locality. It is frequently without merit or justification. Cases in point may include for instance the lack of an Accident and Emergency Department in every hospital, or the clinically necessary centralisation of highly specialist services in one major provider to sustain a critical service which is safe and effective. This can be considered when addressing variation across the NHS.

The term 'postcode lottery' has found more common ground and media attention, where there are decisions by some commissioners either to fund or not fund a new technology, or where an individual has claimed that a certain drug is available in one area but not prescribed in another. This type of variation is harder to explain to the public and should be considered as unwarranted variation.

If all variation were bad, solutions would be easy. The difficulty, according to Mulley (2010) is *'in reducing the bad variation, which reflects the limits of professional knowledge and failures in its application, while preserving the good variation that makes care patient-centred. When we fail, we provide services to patients who don't need or wouldn't choose them while we withhold the same services from people who do or would.'*

This is a fundamental issue for front-line clinicians to address. Are we treating the right patients and are we using the resources in the best way for the population? Is there variation at all? Well, of course there is, and Wennberg's work studying practice variation, using different methods, argued that: *'unwarranted variation in healthcare delivery, which is that variation which cannot be explained on the basis of illness, medical evidence, or patient preference – is ubiquitous.'*

The NHS has been trying to understand variation for some time, but needs to articulate where variation is acceptable and where it is not. This is referred to as unwarranted variation. It is also perhaps the causes of those variations which are most important to understand before we can address unwarranted variation, that prompted the publication of the **NHS Atlas of Variation 2010.**

There is often a simple claim that more resources may help the NHS address unwarranted variation, but do we really know what we currently spend on our services and what more we could do with those resources to extract higher value? Wennberg (2010) claims that additional resource is not the issue and that much healthcare is of questionable value. (This issue was explored in more detail earlier in Chapter 3.)

There is also the significant issue of changing the culture of NHS clinicians, so that they address this issue and accept their part in the redefining of the NHS as a patient-centred service, which outlives the paternal doctor-patient relationship. This will require strong leadership and determined effort from all, starting with the appreciation of variation as an issue, incorporating consideration of understanding unwarranted variation in the basic training for all disciplines.

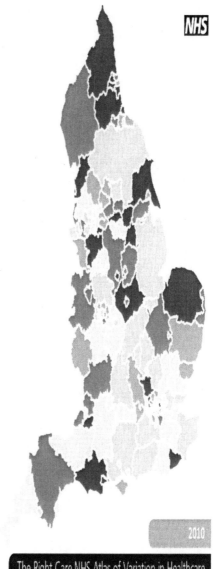

Right Care
The NHS Atlas of
Variation

Addressing un-warranted
variations in healthcare
to improve value

FIGURE 11: COVER OF NHS ATLAS

In this publication, 34 maps across a range of specialties reflect some of the variations in the NHS. It is important to acknowledge that it is highly likely that areas not chosen also have significant variation and the publication of the NHS Atlas of Variation 2010 was only the start. One of the most powerful and inescapable conclusions that has emerged ... **is that physician behaviour is behind much of the variation we experience now.**

However, the publication of this document could be a seen as a defining moment for the NHS. The document stresses the importance of transparency about variations in healthcare services. Its ambition is to engage in a wider conversation about value and how benchmarking performance locally and nationally, will be critical in any strategy that is to be effective at improving quality and reducing cost. More information about the Atlas can be found at www.rightcare.nhs.uk

It is evident that there is considerable variation in referral practice, both within and across Primary Care Trusts and general practices (Starfield 2005).But what can be done once variation is identified? Can more be done about the unwarranted variation that exists in all healthcare economies? One approach to addressing unwarranted variation is to invest more time and effort in shared decision-making, including sound measures to improve outcomes. Measures designed to ensure that decisions are made with the personal knowledge of what the illness, treatment and possible outcomes mean to the patient could create a greater awareness among clinicians and patients of the complexity of decision-making.

General medical practitioners and their community-based teams are well positioned to work with patients and the population, to improve the quality of decisions across a range of illnesses because of their accessibility, their on-going relationships, and their orientation to the whole system rather than just to symptoms and disease.

Primary care clinicians are also well placed to create learning healthcare systems that capture the collective experience of patients, using the evidence about what works for whom, and what is valued by whom, to improve care processes.

Shared decision-making – right care for patients

The principle of 'no decision about me without me' requires all decisions, particularly those in which the patient's values are very important, to be a shared decision, between the patient sitting with you and the clinician. Often clinicians will claim that they are the best advocate for the patient and many of those clinicians claim to have engaged in shared decision making for many years So, if it is not new, why is it causing tension amongst some clinicians?

Well, clinicians have taken the lead in making decisions based on evidence of what is the right thing to do. Throughout the 1990s, evidence-based decision-making became the dominant paradigm, always clearly emphasising that decisions about individual patients should be evidence-based, not evidence-driven, because there are other factors in the decision making process.

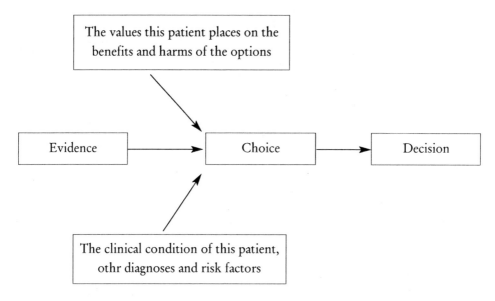

FIGURE 12: A FRAMEWORK ON USING EVIDENCE FOR INDIVIDUAL PATIENTS

The job of the clinician is to relate the evidence to the unique clinical condition of the particular patient, sometimes called personalising evidence, and then to help them relate the evidence to their values through shared decision making.

To pee or not to pee – sex is the question

This may appear to be a strange way of introducing patient decision-making, but let us explore the issue further. Professor Jack Wennberg is the guru of variation in healthcare and has written much on the subject, especially on the importance of really placing patients at the centre of healthcare decisions. In his book *Tracking Medicine – a Researcher's Quest to Understand Health Care (2010)*, Professor Wennberg describes how:

> 'the democratization of the physician-patient relationship – the replacement of delegated decision making by shared decision making and the doctrine of informed consent by a standard of practice based on informed patient choice, represents a transformation in the culture of medicine that will not be easy to achieve.'

As previously noted, there are many clinicians who firmly believe that they aspire to involve the patient at each and every step of the way through the system, offering real *informed* choice about their health, based on the evidence and the interventions or options available to that individual at that time. That is excellent, but, sadly, there are those who still seek to 'direct' or steer the patient, offering little or no choice, and displaying behaviours which retain the 'doctor knows best' attitudes of the service. There are frequent challenges, by clinicians, declaring that the patient often having been given all the options always refers back to the clinician for advice. This is a key part of the positive patient-clinician relationship. But the main issue here is, as a clinician, have you really given the patient all the known information about possible benefits and the potential harm of the intervention? What were the options you made available to, say, the last ten patients you assessed and if they chose to, in what way did you help them navigate through the system?

Common to all assessments of value is the balance between benefit and harm – or the probability of benefit and the probability of harm – and cost. During a recent encounter, Professor Wennberg went on to share a story, with great gentleness, about how an elderly gentleman, faced with a problem of 'nocturnal frequency', was presented with the full information of both the benefits and risks before embarking on invasive surgery. Whilst the benefits of intervention may be that an operation may reduce the frequency of passing water and offer the gentleman more control, the risk of impotence may be too much for that gentleman to bear.

So, shared decision-making is a critical part of a modern healthcare system. Clinicians must remind themselves of the patients' central place in the system and to consider what they bring to the consultation. Furthermore, at a time when resources are limited, developing shared decision-making as a central facet of the NHS, offers another opportunity to increase value, including the opportunity of patients to make informed choices about releasing resources without adversely affecting their health or that of the population.

Clinicians, can all think of the things we would like to do more of. It may be right that we should – for example consider more clinical interventions and operations, or more family-orientated clinics, or a Community Psychiatric Nurse for the elderly to attend more open lunch meetings in support of the Alzheimer's Society. Very often though, many clinicians and front line staff believe that they are already working flat out in a service with ever expanding demand, but with no more resource.

Ask yourself the following questions:

how many things can we think of that you really do not need to do, where no real value is added to the patient care and which is perhaps perceived more of a diktat from the bureaucracy in which you work?

how frequently does a patient return for an outpatient appointment when feeling relatively well and healthy, where the appointment schedule requires the appointment – rather than the progression or deterioration of the condition?

how many patients cannot get to see a specialist clinician because the appointments are already fully booked with routine follow-ups?

what about the home visit by the district nurse when the patient-nurse exchange is really described as being more social than clinical (do not underestimate the role community nurses play in their community), and where risk-averse behaviour is driving the necessity of increasing visits rather than need and better management through informed patient choice?

During these increasingly demanding times, clinicians have to stop and ask: whilst seeing the patients currently in the system, **are we under providing for a number of our patients and over-providing for others?** Or, if we are seeing the right patients, **how could we use our clinical knowledge and skills to innovate and change the way we currently work? Could clinician's help their managers understand the benefits of change**, rather than frequently accepting change from the top down? **Could they innovate in a way which reawakens the spirit,** rather than just being able to muddle through, and do what is expected and not what is required?

It is interesting that some front-line clinicians start to feel a little uncomfortable when reading this, claiming that they always discuss all the alternatives with their patients. That is good, but it's worth challenging whether that it is always true. Do clinician's adopt a process of treating the symptom or condition, and not the patient? **Do we know or understand the values the patient brings to the consultation and intervention?**

Thus, shared decision-making is a vitally important approach to bringing a better balance to the system, to delivering an important step change in the personalisation of healthcare. A personalised approach will take account of the person's preference and the way in which they want to take part in their treatment and care; after all, 'the ambition surely must be to achieve healthcare outcomes that are amongst the best in the world. This can only be realised by involving patients fully in their own care as there may be a tendency for some patients to overestimate benefit and underestimate the risk of healthcare interventions, if they do not have enough information and support to make an informed decision. This can lead to over-use of healthcare in some areas.

Reflecting on many coaching experiences, how easy it can become to ignore the patient during service reviews and focus on the professionals and the system. So, if the system is designed to serve the patient, why does it feel so often that we leave the patient until the end of the discussions, responding in a reactive way, rather than seeking active engagement? There are probably several reasons for this. The first is that we don't always make our population aware of the resources available, or ask our population what the system should look like. Earlier chapters have demonstrated the importance of this and the benefits this can bring.

There are, of course, important issues to consider when thinking about this. Who are the best advocates? Is there a representative group with which we can have a dialogue? How do we prevent a system being designed for those who shout loudest? Might the service they prefer be so complex that we fear the answer, and by not being able to respond to that design, we create an inflexible system? We need to change the relationship the health service has with the public and patients to one of 'co-production', so that we can do the right things safely and effectively. This will not only deliver what our patients need, but will also help us to manage the relentless demand for healthcare within our available resources.

It is evident that the public have not always been included in the debate about the development or design of health services, or the process of resource allocation. Patients are not sufficiently involved or supported in decisions about their healthcare and continue to tell us that they wish to become more involved.

We should be more open and listen, *really listen*, to patient views. There is a very good easy-to-read book by Peter Davies and James Gubb entitled *Putting Patients Last* which describes how, as a business, the NHS continues to forget the patients. One way to address this, in a positive way is through shared decision-making.

7

POPULATION MEDICINE – GENERAL PRACTICE AND CONSULTANT RESPONSIBILITIES IN THE 21ST CENTURY

T he recognition that doctors have responsibilities to the population as well as to the individual patient is increasing both implicitly and explicitly.

General medical practitioners have practised population medicine since 1948, when each was given a defined population for which they were responsible. Hospital clinicians too have population responsibilities, which they recognise and exercise to a greater or lesser extent. But some recent trends in healthcare management have perhaps had the unforeseen consequence of lessening the opportunities for these groups of clinicians to integrate care and retain a focus on population well-being.

Quality of care has been a dominant paradigm for the last three decades. The value of care will be the dominant paradigm in the next three decades. Improving effectiveness, safety, and productivity all contribute to better value care, as does the move to make the patient experience better. The clinician's focus on those issues has been important and needs to continue, but improving quality alone is not enough.

Like quality, the word **'value'** has many meanings and is discussed in Chapter 2. Value in this latter sense relates to the question of how we get the distribution of resources between different patient groups right. As discussed earlier, with programme budgeting, this may be either resource allocation between groups of patients with different types of need, for example mental illness or cancer, *or* within a specialty to patients with different conditions – for example, in a respiratory service, the distribution of resources between asthma, chronic obstructive pulmonary disease, sleep apnoea, interstitial lung disease, and rare conditions. Once the resources have been allocated, the value derived is measured by the health gain – the difference between the benefit and harm – that results from the use of a given resource in any one area of allocation, for example for people with asthma or people with bipolar disorder.

The focus of *quality improvement* has been on the patients referred to a service. But the focus of *value improvement* has to be on the population served by the system, including those people with the disease who are not yet in contact with the service. To maximise value from limited resources, it is essential that all clinicians move toward understanding and developing this concept and adopt a population perspective and responsibility.

How can clinicians promote population health?

Imagine you are a rheumatologist in Tweetshire Royal Infirmary. Last year you saw 346 patients with rheumatoid arthritis. You have worked hard to improve the effectiveness and safety of the service offered, reducing its cost while at the same time concentrating to ensure that each of the 346 patients had a good experience. This is evidence-based, patient-centred, and better quality medicine, all necessary and praiseworthy

However, applying the principles of population medicine, as enabled by training and required by contract, you have to ask how many other people in the Tweetshire County population of 1.5 million have rheumatoid arthritis. By reviewing the Tweetshire prevalence literature and the prescribing patterns of the general practitioners of the county, you estimate that about 2,000 people have rheumatoid arthritis – not all of them diagnosed, and some perhaps wrongly diagnosed. A small survey working with other clinicians allows you to estimate that 400 of those not yet referred would obtain great value from your service

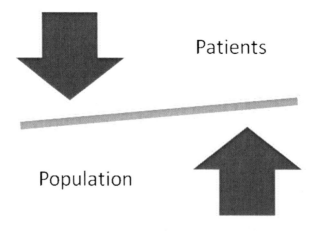

Patients

Population

FIGURE 13: BALANCING THE NEEDS OF PATIENTS VERSUS THE LOCAL POPULATION

Rather than seek extra resources, you do an audit which suggests that 200 of the 346 patients you are already seeing could be looked after by generalists – perhaps with email and telephone support and a clearly defined pathway, expressed through a localised adoption of the Map of Medicine. During the sessions in your working week, which specify your responsibility to improve the health of all people with rheumatoid arthritis, you write an Annual Report on rheumatoid arthritis within your population, working with third sector colleagues. This allows you to compare the population-based performance, using nationally agreed outcomes and standards, with that of the 77 other rheumatoid arthritis services in England. Commissioners have allocated a clearly defined budget for your population service. Not all of it is necessarily under your direct control, because the service is delivered systemically and not bureaucratically, through a network and not a hierarchy.

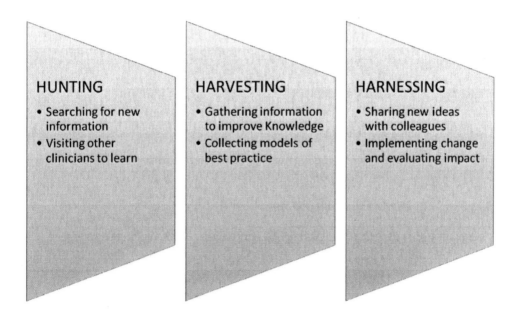

HUNTING
- Searching for new information
- Visiting other clinicians to learn

HARVESTING
- Gathering information to improve Knowledge
- Collecting models of best practice

HARNESSING
- Sharing new ideas with colleagues
- Implementing change and evaluating impact

FIGURE 14:THE 3 H MODEL OF CHANGING PRACTICE

You use the Internet to run the network and offer patients unbiased information. You and your team would feel responsible for all the resources used by the population-based service, and your job description reflects this. Should you also be paid for population-based results?

This may not be such a meaningless remark. Indeed it has been proposed by Mandel (2010) that hospitals could be reimbursed for their impact on populations, not just the subset of the population that happens to have been referred. There is also evidence, Daren, T. *et al.* (2008) that paying generalists, NHS general practitioners, has made *'a substantial contribution to the reduction of inequalities in the efficacy of clinical care'*. Financial incentives, like many invasive procedures, however, can do harm as well as good. It is more important to encourage clinicians, both generalists and specialists, to feel that they are jointly the stewards of the resource with a passion for making the best use of that resource, for the population they serve that matches the passion they bring to their clinical practice with individual patients.

This is the very reason for clinicians to engage and appreciate the positive impact they can have on improving outcomes for their patients and populations. With the added value of well developed and supported clinical input, the commissioning of services for the population can improve quality *and* increase value.

8

A WORLD OF CHANGE: MAKING CLINICAL COMMISSIONING WORK FOR YOU & YOUR POPULATION

T here is no point hiding the fact; change is nearly always difficult to make. It takes us out of our comfort zone by removing or diluting the familiar. It requires additional effort and attention when we are already fully committed to existing responsibilities. By its very nature, change is also disruptive. It usually requires new learning, new ways of working, and quite possibly even new behaviours. Most of all, it is a distraction which potentially requires emotional energy to be re-directed away from the day job.

For these reasons, change is rarely welcome – especially when it feels as though it is forced upon us. And yet, the 60-year story of the National Health Service is one of endless revision, evolution and innovation. The NHS never can stand still. It is instilled with a culture of change, forever re-shaped by different policies, innovation, new clinical practices, clinical research, rising expectations and media scrutiny.

It is one of the ironies of the NHS that this principle of change is ever-present. But there are two other very important constants also: the people who turn to the NHS for care, treatment and support – and the nurses, doctors, physiotherapists, pharmacists and many others who provide it. This precious relationship between patients and clinicians is a golden thread, a source of stability even when the status quo is challenged.

Not surprisingly, quite a responsibility rests on the shoulders of clinicians. More than anyone, they experience the conflicts and uncertainties of the shifting environment in which they work. The way they respond to those challenges is a crucial factor as to whether the NHS continues to advance, or not.

Not all change is necessarily for the best. Even if it is well-intentioned and based on sound evidence, views of it may be tainted if it is imposed rather than developed through collaboration. How often have NHS employees complained about the cost and diversion of re-organisations? But at a time when the National Health Service is said to be undergoing some of the biggest changes since its foundation, there are great opportunities for health professionals at all levels of seniority and influence – opportunities to achieve higher standards, deliver better health outcomes, spread good practice, invent and innovate, forge new partnerships and empower patients more effectively than ever before.

For all of this to be accomplished, there has to be recognition that the opportunity exists at all. Clinicians should be the architects of change, mapping out the terrain, building and shaping the future. As such, they have some important roles to fulfil at:

- **LEADING** – embracing change and ensuring it does become an opportunity for improvement through innovation;
- **RECONCILING** – recognising the tensions and conflicts that arise and not letting them dominate, so that change can be positive;
- **INVOLVING** – engaging with patients as never before both in the choices about their own personal healthcare, in decisions about how money is spent and how wider NHS services are configured.

These are all themes which appear frequently in this book. They help to identify the challenges we face, and the ways we can turn them to advantage.

LEADING – making a difference as clinicians

To react adversely to a difficult situation is to be human. The "fight or flight" reactions kick in as part of our instinctive defence mechanisms. Consider a patient hearing for the first time that they have a very serious or even terminal condition. They will face a whole gamut of emotions: disbelief, fear, anger and then after the initial emotional turmoil, a hunger for knowledge. There may be resignation or despair, and ultimately a steely determination to get through what awaits. It is a sequence of responses articulated by Dr Elisabeth Kübler-Ross (1969) in her "Five Stages of Grief":

- **Denial** – "It can't be me."
- **Anger** – "Why does it have to be me?"
- **Bargaining** – "What if I do this and you do that, to change the situation?"
- **Depression** – "It's really happening, so what's the point?"
- **Acceptance** – "I can't fight it, so I may as well get on with it."

This proposition was originally formulated in connection with the gloomiest of all scenarios, but let's be honest: as a clinician, how many of these responses have you personally experienced, when you have been confronted with a major change or challenge in your work environment or even fresh data sets indicating your performance? It is a natural reaction is to resent such situations; to feel "done to" and not in control; to either actively oppose it, or stage a "sit down protest", adopting a neutral stance which in fact makes the implementation of the change difficult and possibly ineffective.

A side-effect of this resistance is the danger that individual departments or even whole services can be left behind, that their lack of progress actually makes variations across the NHS even greater. On occasions, opposition can even lead to direct conflict between clinical colleagues or different NHS organisations – something to be addressed in the forthcoming section on reconciliation.

Good clinical practice and consensus can mitigate this. All clinicians, regardless of grade or location, need to show leadership by staying in control of their own bit of the world, contributing to the system in which they function by increasing value. After all, they show leadership every day, in the deep and expert knowledge they apply and the decisions they make to help others. This is not about being in charge of teams or holding a position of authority. It means demonstrating personal leadership by taking responsibility, keeping abreast of the latest thinking and implementing it where appropriate, reducing waste and eliminating duplication. Equally, it means shaping new thinking yourself and then sharing it with others so they can adopt it. In this way, change is less likely to be a surprise or imposed. There is a series of simple questions which clinicians can regularly ask them-selves to help with this as follows:

On knowing and implementing best practice:

- How regularly do I take stock of what I do – both the processes I use and the outcomes I achieve?
- How much time do I have for planning or horizon scanning? If I don't have enough, how do I get more?
- When did I last study and implement a piece of relevant good practice from elsewhere?
- Do we as a team get together to discuss and review the quality of what we do?
  On developing a whole population approach:
- How much genuine population-based insight do I have? Do I know how to get more?
- How often do I see patients I know don't need my expertise? What if anything have I done about that?
- Do I seek out patients who I know need my skills and expertise, but I don't see? If not, why not – and how would I do it?
- Do I match resources with demand? Do I even know where to start?
  On being more personally effective:
- What is my relationship like with my manager(s)? Can I improve it?
- When did I last get constructive feedback?
- How often do I get the chance to share my experiences with colleagues?
- What are the irritations and worries in my role? How can I eliminate them?
  On empowering the patient:
- How much genuine involvement do my patients have in shaping their clinical journey? How can I improve it?
- Do I have access to outcomes data for my patients? If not, how do I get it?
- When did I last change something as a result of patient feedback?
- Can I gather my own patient feedback?

Susan Oliver (2006) alludes to the importance of self-enquiry when considering leadership in the NHS:

> To be an effective leader requires a complex mix of attributes, behaviours and skills, but most of all it requires an ability to reflect upon and evaluate yourself. (p38)

In particular, clinicians need to ask for the time and space to seek out best practice and use it to challenge their own way of doing things. Healthcare, whether it be nursing, medicine or other professions, has always had a culture of forward progression, professional learning and personal development. That is a source of great strength. It has driven the massive improvements that we have seen – improvements in identifying diseases, new drugs and technologies, keyhole surgery, genetics, shorter beds stays, stem cells, and so on. Part of that same spirit needs to be harnessed in the day job and engaging in clinical commissioning offers that opportunity.

This need not be delivered independent of others. Indeed, peer support is so important. Such self-examination can be even more effective in teams – particularly if the questions asked lead to a decision to change an established way of doing things. Being proactive and potentially embracing change in this way can protect and enhance the reputation of you and your department with the organisational hierarchy – what Cyert and March (1963) called the "dominant coalition", the people who really run the place – but more importantly, enhance the reputation of your clinical practice with the patients you care for.

There are examples within the NHS where individual clinicians have held a vision and worked with others, to build multi-million pound high-quality services from very small beginnings. In the process, they have broken the mould for the way things are done locally, drawing in colleagues from other sectors and creating a compelling case for change. So what are the triggers that allow this to happen? Here is a reminder of one clinician's recipe for success:

> Existing practice can be quite comfortable, so you do need the right circumstances to make a change. For me, it was quite a large gamble, but it was the right time to try. My personal motivation is being master of my own destiny and doing my best for patients, integrating care not the them and us behaviours I was getting frustrated with. Ultimately, most clinicians want to be good clinicians. What we need now is proper integration of such projects so that the bar is raised overall.

The idea of such a "bottom-up" approach is advocated by John Smythe (2007). He advocates the concept of "co-creation", where the wider workforce can help to shape policy.

In effect, this is leadership that starts at the top, but only really comes to life in the clinical environment. It is in the corporate interest to demonstrate innovation and staff empowerment, to exploit the opportunity. Just look at the success of the NHS Institute releasing time to care: the Productive Series (www.institute.nhs.uk) concept, where NHS Trusts across the country have encouraged nurses and other front line clinical teams to find ways of working more efficiently, to create more time for patient care.

This has spawned many other change schemes such as "Better for You" at Nottingham University Hospitals NHS Trust (www.nuh.nhs.uk). Frontline teams there have been involved in scores of projects to trial, implement and evaluate ideas put forward by both staff and patients. The emphasis may have been on saving money, but as the trust's Chief Executive Peter Homa (2011) said:

> In not one case have we found existing services incapable of improvement. *(p19)*

It is right to celebrate the success of such initiatives, so that what goes well is shared through professional networks. Only in this way can tools and theory be applied to achieve real progress, which in turn is then acknowledged and adopted in other parts of the NHS.

This assumption of personal clinical responsibility is an interesting blend of types of leadership. A transactional "top down" approach can signal a need or desire to change, but the real transformation is achieved through a more democratic, collaborative approach (Burns, 1978). It demonstrates how every individual clinician really can have a role to play. As Susan Oliver (2006) puts it:

> There is an increasing recognition that the wide-ranging changes necessary within the NHS cannot be implemented using a dictatorial management style that enforces change using a 'top down approach'... ...Leadership was seen purely as a management role – yet it is acknowledged now that leaders can be recognized or nominated from within their team for specific tasks and may not necessarily have a role of recognized authority within the organization. Clinicians must have leadership expertise in all settings to implement change based upon good clinical decision making and around a patient-centred approach to care. *(p40)*

When a number of nursing leaders were interviewed to find out what influenced and motivated them, (Antropus and Kitson, 1999), there was

- mention of politics,
- academic reputations,
- corporate factors,
- as well as clinical matters.

But the patient always has to come first. Because of their role, nurses are particularly well placed to draw upon what they learn from patients. A lot of leadership theory is based on the notion that change is largely driven by external factors, such as shifts in national policy.

However, that should not stop clinicians seizing the moment and turning change into an opportunity.

It is not very long ago that Sadie Williams (2004) produced a pretty gloomy assessment of leadership in the NHS and other parts of the public sector:

> ...managers do not seem to be responding to the need for new and more flexible ways of working and thinking. There is also a tension between the emphasis on standards, targets and procedures and the need for creativity and modernisation. There are no rewards for creativity and innovation. *(p26)*

In fact, there are plenty of shining examples of clinical innovation, which we need to harness more widely. Take the thorny issue of rising hospital admissions, with which the NHS is constantly grappling. Research has shown that more than a decade ago, progress was being made (Dusheiko *et al*, 2003) with clinicians taking a direct interest in the design and shape of services. So was the reduction in admissions a result of having responsibility for budgets and being confronted by explicit prices? Why were the gains that had been made not sustained? Those are interesting questions, considering the nature of clinical behaviour during reform. Politics aside, the research does confirm the difference which GPs can make as the gatekeepers of our health system.

When we fast forward to the present day, we find that the pressure has increased. Emergency admissions are now rising at around 9% a year, fuelled by a similar growth in the number of self-referrals to A & E. Emergency admissions are costing more than all planned hospital spells and procedures combined. This elective work is under threat because so much resource – staff, beds and money – is being consumed by the emergency maelstrom. In fact, bed crises are no longer the preserve of winter alone.

So what's causing it? It can't all be down to demographics, can it? Well, bed days for patients aged over 75 rose by 66% in the last 10 years, and now account for more than half of all emergency bed occupancy. Such growth is just not sustainable and as a system, clinicians must work together to identify these patients and co-create more effective pathways and processes for care. This is the only way the NHS will become more effective and patient experience will improve and value increased.

It is, of course, a national issue, but there are significant variations. For a start, not all hospitals admit over 75s at the same rate and clinical commissioning groups are in the prime position to identify and focus on these patients. The patients will be known to many staff, and may well be in communication with a variety of health professionals in both generalist and specialist arenas. But do we stop and assess the situation and ask:

- How many patients are coming into the service?
- What is their route into the service?
- Who is coming into the service?
- Which groups are utilising the majority of the resources?
- Is it effective or even what the patient wants?

There are excellent examples of this happening and when analysis was done in one region (Clay and Longman, 2010), a single general practice stood out among more than 600. The practice's over-75 patients were not only the least likely to attend A & E, but also the least likely to be admitted to hospital. Moreover, there are virtually no patient complaints.

Comparisons with other similar practices confirmed that geography and social conditions could not explain the variation on their own. But this particular practice was an outlier in one other very important way. In the Patient Experience Survey, people are asked how easy they feel it is to speak to a doctor. The proportion of over 75s in this practice who said it was **very** easy to talk to a GP was more than ten percentage points higher than anywhere else in the entire region!

The explanation for this staggering difference is remarkably simple. The practice employs a system which ensures that telephone responses to patient queries are prioritised and happen quickly. Of the 155 calls made to the surgery in a single week, the median response time was 26 minutes. In other words, half of all patients who rang got to speak to a doctor on the phone within half an hour – with no distinction made between "urgent" and "routine" cases.

This was made possible through a review of processes and the introduction and refinement over time of a system which changed working patterns and priorities so that GPs were available to respond quickly when patients called. Often those people only wanted advice. This is an example of shared decision-making in its purest form. Once information was imparted and they were reassured, the patients did not feel the need to go anywhere else – such as the nearest A & E. Think about the issue of cause and effect in this instance?

It's not rocket science, is it? And yet, we know that many patients continue to complain about how hard it is to see their GP. The results of the 2009/10 GP Patient Survey (Ipsos MORI, 2010) showed that while most people are satisfied, significant numbers still say it is difficult to get through on the phone or book an appointment within 48 hours.

The variation in patient experience suggests that not all GPs and practice managers attach the same importance to the issue. Those which have invested modestly in new technology to offer online booking and text reminders say they have reduced the number of patients who miss appointments – a common irritant in primary care. Is it cost, a lack of objective research to confirm the benefits, or an absence of will, which prevents others from following suit?

The practice which has achieved such remarkable results with Doctor First is The Cottage Surgery in the Leicestershire village of Woodhouse Eaves. Its senior partner, Dr Stephen Clay, estimates that if the system was implemented across England, it could save around £1bn in practice costs and a further £1bn in secondary care. He proposed that:

> Doctors have set up systems to protect themselves from the onslaught of patients. We didn't have any more capacity to see more patients in our surgery. So we offer people access to our medical knowledge very quickly, by phone. As a result, 30% more patients have contact with us than the national average. This is about adjusting working patterns to the demands of the day. It doesn't mean you have to work harder, just smarter.

This is pure clinical leadership. Staff identified a situation that required serious investigation and came up with a solution. They re-shaped their organisation and bureaucracy to put the patient first – and in doing so, they found other benefits too. Not only that, they're now introducing the system to others across England (have a look at www.productiveprimary care.co.uk).

This is the sorting of sharing that other parts of the NHS need to emulate. GPs in different parts of the country have developed similar schemes to improve patient access. But they are still in a minority and the spreading of innovation is difficult because of the fragmented nature of the business; every general practice operates autonomously and has its own way of doing things. Those practices which are not proactively seeking out good ideas to try and improve their own service are letting down their patients.

The obvious conclusion from the success of Doctor First is that many patients are going to A & E or other NHS services out of exasperation at not being able to speak to their own family doctor. Or do they genuinely need reassurance? Dr Clay reckons there are five reasons why people attend A & E:

1. They have an injury best dealt with at A & E
2. They have an emergency medical problem best dealt with at hospital
3. They THINK they have an injury best dealt with at A & E
4. They THINK they have emergency medical problem best dealt with at hospital
5. They cannot access a doctor any other way.

What proportion of the entire national A & E workload falls into these last three categories? Think how much value we could gain and how liberated the NHS would be if all those patients could be persuaded to take different courses of action! Of course, it's not as simple as that. Managers and clinicians across the healthcare system have been trying to resolve this issue for years, without success. Could it be that the NHS has forgotten to take an integrated "whole system" approach? Efforts to change patient behaviour have perhaps not focussed enough on ensuring that the alternatives to A & E (GPs and out-of-hours services) are as responsive as they can be and reduce the burden of hospital dependency.

So at this time of heightened change in the NHS, when the financial pressures are huge and responsibility for commissioning is transferring from primary care trusts to clinical commissioning groups, it is clinicians who are best-placed to show leadership – something advocated by the NHS Institute for Innovation and Improvement:

> Clinicians are the public face of the organisation. They may remain in the same post for many years and have considerable experience of the NHS. This gives them a wealth of knowledge about the strengths and weaknesses of the system. The decisions and actions they take have a direct bearing on the use of the organisation's resources.

The lack of breathing space is a challenge for all clinicians. But the message is that clinical colleagues cannot afford to ignore opportunities to improve what they do:

> Most doctors don't have the time to think ahead because they're too busy fire fighting. Most GPs would say they're stressed and can't do any more than they do. We discovered there were lots of things we did that we didn't need to do. It's such a tiny effort compared to the gain it gives you.

Significant benefits for the wider system can result from comparatively modest innovation at a local level. But the full potential of such initiatives can only be fully reached if all the innovators are prepared to celebrate and share what they've achieved, including both pitfalls and benefits. Further achievement will follow when clinicians come together across professional networks and organisational boundaries, in pursuit of greater productivity, better outcomes and consistent standards.

This is crucial if the NHS is to succeed in dealing with the challenges it faces – reconciling emotional responses with rational choices, and system-wide thinking with organisational loyalties. It is this requirement for reconciliation which I want to address in the next section.

RECONCILING – recognising the tensions and not letting them dominate

Clinicians are used to making decisions. They face and answer scores of questions every day. What is the right diagnosis here? Are drugs or treatment needed, and what sort? Do I need a second opinion – if so, where from? When do I need to review this case? Should I involve social services or other agencies? To which patient do I give the single bed available? Does this person require another home visit? And so on.

Clinical decision-making is a rational business. The evidence is gathered and assessed; options are considered; risks and benefits evaluated; the decision is made, communicated and implemented. It usually requires only minutes, but may take weeks if the right evidence is difficult to obtain. Nevertheless, the nature of the process is consistent, based as it is on the objective analysis of data through the application of knowledge.

In this activity, clinicians are at their most effective. It is what they are trained for, where they are confident, and why they are doing the great job they do. The head is very much in control. However, we know life is not that simple. Clinicians are human beings, with emotions which have a habit of getting in the way! In our everyday world this happens all the time. The decisions we make are influenced by whims and feelings, as well as logic. Thus we care what colour of car we buy, we choose our holidays carefully, and buy a particular type of sandwich for lunch because we happen to fancy it that day. This is who we are – heart and head operating in tandem.

Health professionals may not think they draw on these emotions for their clinical decision-making, but they are always there below the surface. At times of change, tension and conflict at work, the emotions can re-emerge. When that happens, there is a real danger that the shift in balance between head and heart may affect the decisions that are made, potentially compromising delivery of the right patient care. Let's look at some of the circumstances in which these tensions can arise:

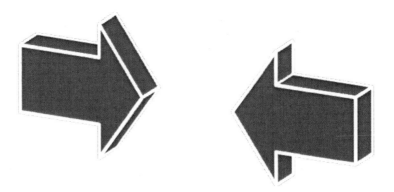

FIGURE 15: HEAD AND HEART TENSIONS

1. Commissioner v provider
2. Primary care v secondary care
3. Managers v clinicians
4. Organisations v individuals
5. Cost v value
6. Patient v population
7. National v local
8. Multiple tensions (any combination of the above)

1 Commissioner v provider

Clinicians who commission services approach issues differently from those who are entirely focussed on delivering the services. They have to balance a myriad of competing demands on the resources and budgets for which they are responsible, with the objectives of meeting all health needs and improving outcomes. They stand on the hill top and view the entire health care landscape.

Clinicians who solely deliver care inevitably concentrate on their patients and the immediate environment in which they operate – whether that is a general practice, a physiotherapy department in a community hospital or a clinical specialism in a specialist hospital. They tend to be fiercely passionate about that world, reacting with hostility to any perceived threat. In such situations their response is an emotional one; and in the reformed NHS, it will be those clinicians who commission; perhaps creating a new level of clinical conflict. Front line clinicians complain about service variation, or "postcode lotteries" as the public do, if they have legitimate concerns. But to see this issue for what it is, those clinicians have to engage with commissioners in the decision-making on a rational level – presenting outcome-based, best practice evidence to win the argument.

Take, for instance, moves in some areas to change referral thresholds for hip and knee replacements. In some cases, it is commissioners who want to eradicate variations in the criteria used by neighbouring acute trusts. In doing so, they may save some money. Orthopaedic surgeons perceive the change as rationing and complain loudly that "their patients" will suffer if they have to wait longer for their operations. This is not a promising position from which to achieve a clinical consensus, but both parties have a logical claim to the moral high ground.

It is essential that all parties should play an active part in such debates, to ensure that decisions are collective and taken on the basis of all the relevant evidence. Everyone must pull in the same direction rather than as separate bureaucracies and cultures:

1. **People who invest in health services want –**
   Value, Allocative Efficiency, Equity, Sustainability

2. **People who provide health services want –**
   Quality, Technical Efficiency, Good patient experience

The removal of unwarranted variation is just as important in primary care. Clinical Commissioning Groups are already proactively challenging and supporting those practices which appear to be referring or prescribing more than their peers. Not all GPs will be receptive to this sort of debate. General practice has been built on operational independence. Helman (2002) talks of the multiplicity of sub-cultures in practices, whose very strength lies in their connections with their own specific local communities. Marshall *et al* (2002) describe this historic independence as undermining the principle of collective responsibility.

As a result, there is tension between GPs who only want to treat their registered patients, and their colleagues who are taking a population perspective through a more active role in commissioning, assessing how resources can be best used for the registered and non-registered population. Having responsibility for commissioning does influence clinical behaviour and the skilled clinician must find a way of harmonising these two dimensions.

2   Primary care v secondary care

By their very nature, primary and secondary care clinicians do different things. The former are generalists, the latter tend to be specialists. Primary care is very local and community-based. Secondary care draws patients from a much wider area to a central hospital site. But there are specialists functioning very effectively in primary care settings, so it is important not to think only of the buildings or organisations, but rather, the system and network.

Each has its areas of strength and expertise and together they integrate. It is important for clinicians to remember where they fit into the wider system, so that they can identify and neutralise the possible areas of contention. The configuring of urgent care services is a good example of this. Not all A & E consultants are comfortable with the move towards having a primary care clinician's presence in their departments. GPs see the generalist approach of primary care triage as a way of avoiding harm and excessive interventions or over-investigation and unnecessary admissions.

Both sides are right. It just needs working out a shift in language. By focussing on best practice and the needs of the patient by delivering properly integrated care pathways, the two groups can work together in harmony. However, Professor Jack Wennberg, a pioneer of work on clinical variation in the United States, recognises that here, there are major cultural obstacles to be overcome:

> You have to have an integrated service in which primary care and specialists work as a team and that's one of the problems that I think I have seen here in the UK, is that there is a cultural chasm between hospital-based specialists and the primary care physicians. We need to break that down somehow.

3 Managers v clinicians

The so-called divide between managers and clinicians has long been a common theme in the NHS. The stakes have been raised by the successive Governments with a clear implication that excess bureaucracy is undermining the effectiveness of the health service; hence the avowed intent to reduce the number of "pen-pushers". This sort of language perpetuates a potentially destructive "them and us" culture, where clinicians complain that managers hinder their work without always making a genuine effort to understand.

The development of Clinical commissioning creates a new dynamic in this regard. Historically, virtually all clinicians have been able to blame invisible people in suits for some of the NHS's shortcomings ("we'd love to give you that expensive drug, but the health authority/primary care trust won't let us"). Now it will be GPs and other clinical colleagues who will be clearly responsible and accountable for advocating such policies rather than criticising them. The clinicians will be a leading part of the system of management they may previously have criticised. As such, they have the critical role of engaging early in the commissioning debate to shape the system for their population.

This tension between management and leadership is a universal theme. Parry and Proctor-Thomson (2003) explored it in New Zealand, but the issues are the same. Clinicians do not want to see themselves as managers. Leadership is a much more attractive label – which is fine, because leadership is what is needed.

4 Cost v value

The new emphasis on "value" as a driving force in the NHS (where cost and quality are considered together) should help to resolve some of the tensions between financial balance and clinical effectiveness, though it may take time. The cost improvement programmes now in place will be hard to deliver, and contract negotiations between commissioners and providers are tougher than they have ever been. The whole QIPP concept (Quality, Innovation, Productivity, Prevention) is encouraging clinicians to review the way they do things, but there is a significant risk that changes designed to achieve improved value will be interpreted as a Trojan horse for cuts.

This book has offered programme budgeting as a real opportunity for clinicians to show their true worth at a time when budgets are stretched. Making the money go further and improving patient outcomes are not incompatible objectives. But it does require enlightened dialogue across the system – and a preparedness to be open-minded by accepting and acting upon data which demonstrates poor value. Evidence of unwarranted variation can be difficult for services which effectively have to admit they have not been performing as well as they could.

5   Patient v population

Here perhaps is the biggest challenge for clinical commissioning groups. Historically, it has been commissioners and public health professionals who have been responsible for identifying and planning for the health needs of the wider population, including ensuring a system and services for those individuals not registered with a general practitioner. Front line clinicians, meanwhile, devote their energies to the individual patients they see every day. Quite rightly, their time is spent focussing on the cases alongside of them; other people not in the health care system may not receive any help, even if they have more pressing needs.

There is a clear mismatch here which needs addressing through changes in both commissioning and service provision. A move to programme budgeting has to be the answer, where the front line clinicians support commissioners in shaping the systems to deliver truly integrated services. Resource can then be allocated according to the wider population need, rather than being spent merely on what walks through the consulting room door. Programme budgeting can lead to greater equity, more coherent care pathways, and therefore greater consistency in quality and accessibility. The suggestion has been to compare the NHS approach with that of the big supermarkets, which would never turn a customer away:

> If you go into Tesco, you get exactly the same service, whether you are starving hungry and have no food in the house, or whether you're just popping in to top up the cupboards. GPs are providing a fantastic service to the few people they see a lot – but what about all the rest? Some get a lousy service, or no service at all.

This will require many clinicians to change their thinking and working culture. The NHS needs more recognition that there can be better ways of doing what's best for patients. But there is also a responsibility on the NHS to ensure that such developments are not left so isolated that their benefits to the wider population are limited.

6   National v local

A focus on unwarranted variation necessitates comparisons. Benchmarking is an increasingly important tool is this respect. Front line clinicians have to be receptive to it and not view it as a threat. It is very easy in such circumstances to become defensive and let the heart rule the head. As one surgeon puts it:

> We're all very fired up about providing the very best for our patients. The trouble is, we don't always know what that is. There's so much evidence that it can get very confusing, and different interpretations of it can be a cause of variation.
>
> So the evidence needs to be readily available and easily digestible. We have to tell consultants how their teams are performing, through comparison. That may be painful for the clinicians at the bottom of the table, but if I was a patient I am not sure that I would want to go to them.

The NHS has always had to deal with the tensions created by being a **national** health service with local decision-making. Local autonomy has to be a good concept, where clinicians are empowered to respond to the particular needs and circumstances of their patients. That is the purpose behind Joint Strategic Needs Assessments, where public health professionals gather and share detailed knowledge about the local population's state of health.

However, as soon as things are done differently at a local level, variation creeps in and as previously stated, not all variation is bad. There are systems in place to try and ensure it is the right sort of variation, but they are not perfect. For example, commissioners rely on guidance from the National Institute for Health and Clinical Excellence (NICE) to help steer them through the moral minefield of expensive drugs and procedures – effectively using the guidance not to fund them locally.

The role of NICE typifies the dilemma faced by the health service on a daily basis. Whether to fund a brief extension of a dying patient's life is a hugely emotive issue. Clinicians acting as the patient's advocate in such circumstances are inevitably drawn into the tug-of-war between head and heart. These tensions are not helped by obvious inconsistencies in the way some policies are applied. Benchmarking, programme budgeting and a reliance on objective data have to play an increasingly central role in ensuring that such variations are valid.

7   Multiple tensions

These different layers of tension illustrate how the professional and personal relationships that bind the NHS together are complex and inter-woven. Therefore there can often be multiple sources of stress at the same time. Clinicians may find themselves being pulled in several different directions at once – making the head v heart conflict even harder to manage.

This is particularly evident during major service re-design. This is a key issue for forming Clinical Commissioning Groups, but one which can be delivered so much better if the complexities of the service are understood from the outset.

Picture the scene. An acute hospital trust is split across two sites some distance apart, with an Accident and Emergency department at both. Support services at the smaller site are limited, patient numbers are comparatively low, and medical staffing levels are far from ideal. Concerns about the viability of the service are growing, on grounds of patient safety, the cost of using locums to fill the medical rotas and the value to the tax payer.

Then new national standards on treatment for heart attack and stroke are adopted, which the smaller site will never be able to meet. Even if millions of pounds were available to develop the right services (and of course, they're not), patient numbers would still be unfeasibly low and the wider hospital network would be destabilised.

The Clinical Commissioning Group, working with the hospital Trust, discusses its concerns and concludes that the smaller A & E unit no longer looks viable and initiates a major service review. The review quickly starts to question the future of some other services on the smaller site. This standpoint is stoutly supported by GPs in the CCG, who see an exciting opportunity to develop a portfolio of services much more based on generalist and community care.

Suddenly the consensus between clinical commissioners and the hospital Trust is broken. Hospital clinicians whose services could be closed or downsized vow to fight any change and start leaking unsavoury and potentially damaging material to the media and local politicians. They have heated debates with some of the local GPs. Struggling to keep all its staff on board and alarmed at the thought that wider changes could lead to a significant loss of income, the provider trust pulls back from full co-operation with the review. But that stance worries the Trust's A & E consultants, who are still anxious about patient safety. In any case, the review is already in the public domain. Protest petitions are circulating, questions are being asked in Parliament and a "Stop The Cuts" campaign by the local paper is gathering momentum. The PCT has to try and proceed with a full public consultation on legitimate issues, without there being any sort of clinical consensus about the way forward.

It's not a happy picture, is it?

What started out as a fully reasoned and rational approach to a difficult problem has degenerated into a free-for-all, where the original rationale has been swamped by a tidal wave of emotions and conflicting loyalties. A wide range of tensions is in play – commissioners against providers, primary care against secondary care, managers against clinicians, organisations against individuals, cost against value, national guidelines against local circumstances. The result is an outbreak of the "tribalism" which Beattie (1995) alluded to when he considered how professional boundaries can influence behaviour. Such a scenario may seem extreme, but many elements of this fictitious story will ring true with people working in various parts of the NHS.

However, it doesn't have to be like this. Reviewing the hypothetical case study reveals that safety issues need to be addressed, so some change is inevitable. That does create real opportunities for integration and for clinicians to work together to re-shape whole pathways for the better. The provider Trust fully engaged can develop new outreach services and integrated care packages to retain its part in the local health system. Stroke and heart patients taken elsewhere for emergency treatment could return for recovery and rehabilitation by community teams hosted by the hospital. The solutions are there. But it requires imagination, courage and innovation from all concerned. Above all, everyone must remember that patient safety and needs always come first.

Of course, there is no magic formula for guaranteeing that such situations won't arise. Indeed, in advocating clinical engagement in decision-making, the NHS Institute for Innovation & Improvement acknowledges that there may be conflict:

> Clinicians have a professional responsibility to their patients, and are answerable to their regulatory bodies...They also have a responsibility to their employing organisation, but regard this as secondary to their professional responsibilities.

> When the organisation proposes process or clinical change which is contrary to that expected by their professional bodies, it can cause conflict. This is why clinicians should be part of every change process. (NHS Inst.)

But conflicts are less likely if a critical mass of clinicians is demonstrating the personal leadership already discussed in this book, putting the wider needs of the patient population first. The construction of integrated pathways will naturally lead to collaboration between primary and secondary care, generalists and specialists, commissioners and providers. This enables professional relationships to develop, trust to build and knowledge to be shared.

So how do we develop the right culture in the NHS for more of this cross-collaboration to flourish? Woodard (2007) provides some excellent insights on establishing successful working across organisational boundaries – starting with the need for backing from the very top, supported by adequate time and resources. The strategic approach to health care planning and provision needs to become part of the working routine:

> To improve efficiency, organisations need to work differently and more intelligently. Working across organisational boundaries makes sense – outcomes can be achieved that would not be feasible for one individual or organisation alone and significant efficiencies can be gained.
>
> Partnerships can enhance individual and organisational success through more effective problem solving, improved adaptation to change, increased efficiency and improved patient care. (p4)

Greater efficiency and improved patient outcomes are only two of the benefits of inter-organisational working. It also offers new perspectives on the whole patient journey, supports benchmarking, aids personal development, provides opportunities to try new things out without fear of failure, and strengthens communication.

In bringing together people from different organisations, Woodard (2007) describes how consideration needs to be given to the distinctive roles each individual will play. This will help to ensure an optimum mix of skills and interests:

- Providers of specific knowledge (eg clinical specialists)
- Those who can bridge the gap between clinical and managerial agendas
- Boundary spanners, whose existing roles make them well placed to bring different organisations and teams together (eg established leads of clinical networks)
- Clinical champions (clinicians who will influence other clinicians).

Groups of clinicians will be able to work together more effectively increasing value if they recognise that there is common ground. It is just a question of finding it. Focussing on the hard evidence – in other words, adopting a rational rather than an emotional approach – is a good place to start.

Thinking strategically helps with this, as it is the more localised specific issues which tend to arouse most emotion. If all clinicians adopt the population-based approach, they are more able to engage with commissioners on a strategic level, playing a meaningful role in the re-design of pathways and services. It is expecting too much for there never to be tensions, but there will be less risk of conflict if all clinicians are able to stand on the hill top, seeing the bigger "joined up" picture.

However, once the clinicians have established a population-wide perspective, they then have to involve the population itself – and when patients and public are brought into play, the battle for hearts and minds becomes even more complex.

INVOLVING – embracing patient empowerment

The NHS has come a long way in how seriously it takes the issue of patient and public engagement. Complex structures and processes have been created to support this. Foundation Trusts and even some PCTs have public membership schemes, Patient and Public Involvement (PPI) committees, and lay representation at Board level. An increasing number of general practices have Patient Participation Groups. We also have an NHS Constitution enshrining patients' rights in law.

But people want a bigger say – or rather, they want a **meaningful** say, where their input can be demonstrably proved to have influenced the way the NHS works. After all, one of the drivers of increasing demands on the health service is rising patient and public expectation, so clinicians should be listening. PPI can no longer be tokenistic. But in its guidance "Real Involvement", the Department of Health (2008) explains the extent of the challenge:

> There is scant evidence to show that involvement activity is stitched into all the strands of NHS organisations' work, including their decision-making processes; of how organisations have listened and responded to what users have told them; or of how health services have been shaped according to the needs and preferences of users. *(p10)*

The NHS Alliance (2010) identifies three main benefits for the NHS of involving the public:

1. Improved service quality and safety
2. Lower costs and improved health – better 'value'
3. Renewed trust and stronger communities.

Nevertheless, weaknesses and uncertainties persist in some parts of the NHS about when to involve service users, and on what terms. Are they genuinely being consulted or just ticking a box? Are patients being led to believe they can change something which is non-negotiable? The Real Involvement document offers the "involvement continuum" as a tool to aid decisions about what degree of engagement is really wanted.

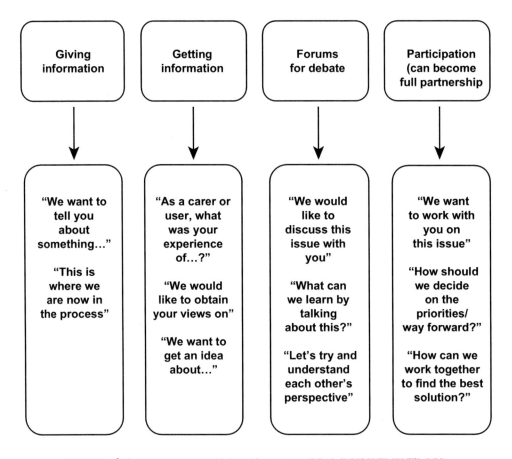

FIGURE 16:THE INVOLVEMENT CONTINUUM, ("REAL INVOLVEMENT", P70)

Legitimate patient and public engagement needs to happen on three levels, and in all of them clinicians have a central role:

1. Individual level: direct interaction with service users so that they can play a full and informed role in decisions about their care.
2. Service level: systematic collection of patient experience data to respond to concerns, maintain or improve standards, and guide commissioning.
3. Strategic level: proactive gathering of relevant public opinion and insight when services are being planned or change is being considered.

The "onion ring" methodology of stakeholder mapping demonstrates how relationships with service users can change, according to the context of the engagement being undertaken. The diagrams that follow in each section show the layers of separation between an individual patient and those seeking engagement and information; the greater the separation, the more difficult it can be for there to be genuine understanding on both sides. The panel to the right of each diagram indicates the information that is wanted by each party.

Individual engagement

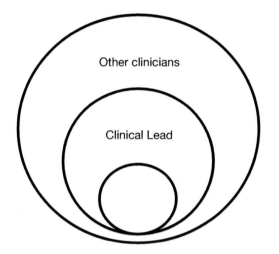

DATA SOUGHT

Patient
Diagnosis, treatment
options and probabilities

Clinical Lead
(Primarily responsible
for patient

FIGURE 17: ON INDIVIDUAL PATIENT ENGAGEMENT

Individual engagement is about a clinician's direct contact with their patient. Here the relationship is strong and immediate. Other clinicians may at some point have dealings with the patient, but the original clinician is best-placed to ensure a real dialogue takes place.

In an NHS where shared decision-making should be paramount and the patriarchal attitude of "doctor knows best" is consigned to history, this two-way conversation really matters if treatment is to be genuinely personalised to meet individual need and preference. Patients can only make informed decisions about their healthcare if real effort has been made to tell them everything they need to know. The input from each side is of equal merit, as Professor Annette O'Connor (2011) explains:

> There are two experts in the relationship; the expert clinician who judges what's wrong, makes a diagnosis... and determines for this patient that there is a range of medically reasonable options, explains the benefits and harms of those options and the probabilities and numbers attached to that and the scientific uncertainties. The role of the patient is to explain their personal situation in relation to these options, as well as to indicate which of the benefits, harms and scientific uncertainties matter most to them in determining treatments.

> We have learned the clinicians are not very good at judging what matters most to patients, they have to ask. You have to ask, and it has to be a dialogue.

There will be times when the information for patients to consider is substantial, and the ensuing decisions about treatment options far from straightforward. Clinicians need to ensure that they are able to adapt their style of communication to be at their most supportive. This includes being able to offer decision support aids – structured materials (both printed and online) which guide patients through the choices they face. The Picker Institute, which has been involved in the piloting of decision-making aids, has recommendations about what they should contain and when they should be used:

Elements for inclusion

- Tailored information about medical conditions and treatment options
- Information about outcomes, benefits and risks, including probabilities
- Materials to help patients explore and articulate what is most important for them
- Other patients' experience of the same situation/decisions
- Information and exercises to prepare patients for an active role in decision-making.

Times when aids to be used

- Treatment options are difficult to compare – eg different outcomes or complications
- Trade-offs – eg short term v long term
- Small risk of a very bad outcome
- Options are all very similar in terms of outcome, risk etc
- Patient has strong priority to achieve a particular outcome or avoid a particular risk.

The provision of such aids is one example of how far the NHS will have to raise its game in the new "information revolution". All patients need to have ready access to details of services and treatment options, the performance of those services and what other patients think about them. The information needs to be simple to understand and well signposted so that it is also easy to find. The scale of the task this presents to all parts of the NHS –

from individual surgeries to large trusts and clinical commissioning groups – is not to be under-estimated. But it needs to be done, and clinicians have to be instrumental in making it happen. Then the strength of the individual engagement they have with their patients will be reflected in other parts of the system.

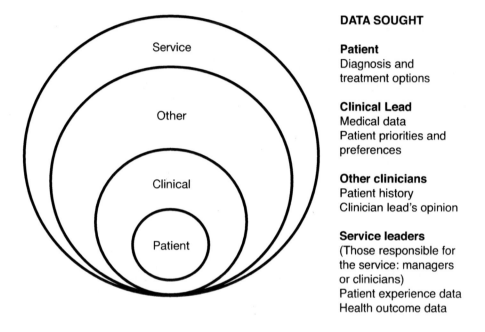

DATA SOUGHT

Patient
Diagnosis and
treatment options

Clinical Lead
Medical data
Patient priorities and
preferences

Other clinicians
Patient history
Clinician lead's opinion

Service leaders
(Those responsible for
the service: managers
or clinicians)
Patient experience data
Health outcome data

FIGURE 18: SERVICE-BASED ENGAGEMENT

At a wider service level, information exchanges with the patient become more remote and strategic. The patient retains the strong relationship with their lead clinician, which has developed through intense contact and dialogue. However, when they are asked to give an opinion on the service, the request usually comes from another part of the organisation. The patient may well give an honest opinion, but rarely with any real sense of how or if it will be used to benefit others.

This can be a weakness in the gathering of patient experience data. It is much more powerful if the request for information comes from the immediate clinical team. It strengthens the patient's connection with the process and makes it real. The process can become even more meaningful if clinicians make the effort to display the results of patient experience data where it can be seen by others. It strengthens the belief of respondents that their views will be heard – particularly if improvements can be demonstrated.

Indeed, all clinical teams should ask themselves if there are gaps in their knowledge which additional patient feedback could fill. Often, insight about care pathways comes from small groups of patient representatives who are well-informed but do not fully reflect the wider population. It is far more meaningful to engage routinely with patients while they are still on their care journey – and as the onion ring diagram demonstrates, clinicians are best-placed to do that. Patient and public involvement can be seen as a chore, but not if it is embedded in daily activity. The Department of Health's "Real Involvement" guidance alludes to this:

> A high-performing organisation does not see involvement as an isolated activity or a hoop to jump through. It sees its users as a valuable source of information, who are able to provide an insight into their needs and wants, and feedback on their experiences...(p27)

Impressions of the NHS are shaped by personal experience – how people have been treated as human beings rather than as patients. It is as much about the attitude of the receptionist, the time spent waiting and the tastiness of the food, as it is about the quality of health care. Clinicians need to have ownership of this data because it can help them to remember the customer service elements of their role. GPs can happily boast about having appointments available every day, but it is not surprising they are under-used if the telephone system is antiquated and people cannot get through. In those circumstances, the practice's reputation will be poor.

Using patient experience data for service design is a powerful tool. All it requires is for clinical teams to hear what patients are saying and act upon it. The NHS Institute for Innovation and Improvement has gathered some inspiring examples of how powerful the insight gathered can be in its simplicity – such as the difficulties faced by fractured neck of femur patients in South Tees because the toilet roll holder was attached to the wall on their weaker side; or the frustration of long-standing renal patients in Wigan who were constantly having to re-acquaint new staff about their circumstances and preferences. A patient-held care plan solved that problem. In these cases, clinical staff showed a commitment to providing a better experience for their patients. Involvement is a core part of service improvement, not an add-on, as Boyle and Harris (2009) explain:

> The people who are currently defined as users, clients or patients provide the vital ingredients which allow public service professionals to be effective. (p11)

At a service level, patient feedback plays another important role. Fran Woodard (2007) points out how service users are best-placed to highlight where care pathways have become disjoined through loose connections or inadequate communication between organisations. Often it is the poor co-ordination of health care which leads to complaints or ineffective care. This is why it can be good practice for different NHS agencies to share feedback data from those patients who cross organisational boundaries.

Therefore clinical teams should ask themselves whether they want to take direct responsibility for the gathering and application of patient feedback about their service. This can be done through printed questionnaires, online surveys, face-to-face, or by focus groups. Showing patients how the resulting information has been used for their benefit can only enhance public confidence in the service.

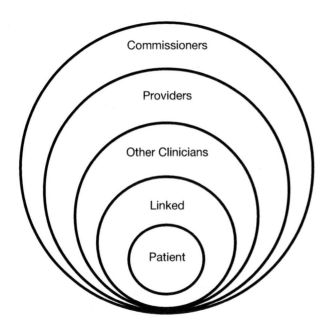

DATA SOUGHT

Patient
Diagnosis, treatment options
Personal impact of any
service change

Linked Clinicians
(Also involved in the
patient's care)
Data about patient
Data on service proposals
Impact of possible change
Views of other clinicians
+ patients

Other clinicians
(In service but not
involved in the patient's care)
Data on service proposals
Impact of possible change
Views of other clinicians
+ patients

Provider Organisations
Corporate impact of change
Views of other clinicians
+ patients
Views of wider public
+ politicians

Commissioners
Views of all parties –
patients, public, partners,
clinicians, politicians

FIGURE 19: STRATEGIC ENGAGEMENT

Strategic engagement can be the most difficult of all to do well. It is primarily undertaken by commissioning organisations to inform decisions about service re-design or disinvestment – either through ongoing structured lay involvement, or through tailored public consultation required by law.

This form of engagement is difficult for two main reasons: the context in which it happens, and the distance between those leading the engagement and the people whose views are being sought.

Context

The issue of why change is rarely welcomed has been discussed, no matter how compelling the reasons for it. When change is proposed to any part of the health service, there will always be people who want to protect the status quo. The staunchest defenders will often be the patients and families who have had a good experience of the service.

Public affection for the NHS is deep-rooted in any case (after all, everyone uses it), and this comes to the fore when a threat is perceived to something that has strong local ownership. Bricks and mortar become symbols of the service. Hence powerful emotions are aroused by consultations which raise the prospect of closing a ward or clinic – let alone an entire emergency department. The sense of loss can be overwhelming, leading to feelings of victimisation ("Why our bit of the NHS?") and even paranoia ("They really want to shut the whole hospital but don't want to admit it").

To some extent, this is inevitable. Our view of the NHS is empirical, based on what we see and experience. We are not interested in organisational shape or systems, but what the NHS does for us and our loved-ones. This explains why strategic engagement can generate particularly powerful conflicts between head and heart. People often understand and accept the rationale for decisions on a theoretical level, and even financially-driven service change. But they react differently when the implications are practical and directly relevant. Even the fear of that personal impact is enough to generate negativity, and this is nearly always strong enough to override the logical response. When arguments for change are presented in the rather sterile context of projected patient flows, business cases and clinical pathways, it is understandable when the public want to remind the NHS that they are real people, not numbers on a page.

Distance

This emotional attachment to services and the people who deliver them contrasts sharply with the role and profile of NHS commissioners. The onion ring diagram demonstrates how they are so far removed from the patients' world as to be virtually invisible. It is as if commissioners and patients are looking down the same telescope – but from different ends.

Many PCTs which have measured public awareness of their existence and role have only achieved percentage recognition rates in single figures. There is a risk that commissioning organisations only enter the consciousness of the local community when they are seen to have bad news to impart – such as an unwelcome service change.

This presents a big challenge for the new Clinical Commissioning Groups – but also opportunities. This book suggested that when controversy arises, there has been a temptation for clinicians to hide behind other clinicians and managers rather than be seen "on the wrong side". In their new commissioning role, some GPs will be much more obvious in the decision-making firing line. It can require moral courage. Those doctors who have been medical directors of primary care trusts can pay witness to the discomfort and even opprobrium this can bring.

And yet, no one is better-placed than front-line clinicians to have a meaningful dialogue with the patients they work with every day. Because of this direct relationship with service users, clinicians who can harness and convey their passion for a particular standpoint are a powerfully persuasive force. Passion is an important word here. Clinicians who articulate a case for service change usually do so on rational grounds, raising the risk of disconnection with the wider public and suspicion about motives ("What's in it for them, have they been bought off?").

The trick is to use both heart and mind by remembering to focus on the patient and the human consequences. Clinicians are well equipped for strategic engagement because they draw upon their built-in empathy for those in their care. In one service review which involved directing more patients to general practice, people were sceptical because of perceived problems about access and waiting times for appointments. The issue became political and few GPs showed any willingness to be questioned at public meetings. The one who did attend explained the financial sacrifice he had made to recruit an additional nurse to meet demand. He spoke with wit, emotion and a clear commitment to his patients. By the end of the meeting, he was a paragon of virtue in the eyes of the audience. Other practices in the area had also made efforts to improve access to their patients. But they were nervous about engaging with the public in an environment they weren't used to. The opportunity to explain what they were doing was lost. The residual impression in the public's mind was that they were somehow second-best.

This is why all clinicians need to understand the importance of patient and public involvement – what the NHS's obligations are, what PPI can contribute, and how to do it well.

Doing engagement well

Designing and delivering high-quality health care is complex. It is more important than ever before that the NHS gets it right – not least, because the public expect nothing less. Effective public engagement is needed to ensure that services are of the right standard and meeting need. But previous poor engagement has made the public cynical about consultation. Too often they are presented with something which looks very much like a fait accompli, because there is no genuine dialogue. The impression is that the NHS is not listening and does not really want to.

The principle of "nothing about me without me" is now enshrined in the NHS Constitution. Many clinicians have embraced this refreshed relationship – sharing information and knowledge to help patients arrive at a decision which suits them. So how do we take such practice and make it work at a "system" level?

The first thing to remember is that the idea of the public having a say in what the NHS does is non-negotiable, particularly where change is concerned. In these circumstances, the requirements are statutory (Real Involvement, 2008). Section 242 of the NHS Act 2006 states that through consultation, information or other means, service users must be involved in:

a) the planning of the provision of those services,
b) the development and consideration of proposals for changes in the way those services are provided, and
c) decisions to be made by that body affecting the operation of those services.

The Government's Code of Practice on Consultation (Cabinet Office, 2005) says that "formal consultation should not be entered into lightly". There are strict rules and taxing audit trails that need to be applied, not least, the Government's four new 'tests' through which service configurations have to demonstrate:

1. Support from GP commissioners (clinical engagement)
2. Strengthened public and patient engagement
3. Clarity on the clinical evidence base
4. Consistency with current and prospective patient choice

Sometimes the scale of what is being proposed is such that consultation is the only option. When that happens, there are elements to include and traps to avoid:

DO:

- Involve service users at the earliest possible stage, long before the formal consultation period. They can help to establish the key principles to be addressed and identify the most contentious areas.
- Keep an open mind and be prepared to change plans. Responsiveness is always appreciated by the public.
- Always offer legitimate options for consideration. The public will see through a lack of choice.
- Ensure the reasons for change are clear and compelling. What are the benefits? Withdrawing a service for operational convenience is not a persuasive argument.
- Make it as easy as possible for everyone to have a say. That means using a range of communication channels and reaching out to every part of the community.
- Be proactive in countering false and scurrilous rumours. They always emerge in times of controversy.
- Report back after consultation so the public know how their views have shaped what is decided. You have to be able to demonstrate a connection if change is to be accepted.

DON'T:

- Under-estimate the amount of time, planning, effort and resource that is needed to do consultation well – or the importance of adequate support from communications and engagement specialists.
- Come to full and final agreement about care pathways before consultation. Otherwise you will present an entrenched position.
- Rule out someone coming up with a better idea than yours. If that happens, be prepared to embrace it.
- Hide difficult issues. They will always emerge. In any case, people expect transparency. For example, if the service is unaffordable, say so. But be aware that the public may still prefer that service to be retained at the expense of something else.

- Ignore the contribution of other NHS staff. After all, they are potential service users and they also provide insights other patients may not.
- Under-estimate the strength of feeling aroused by issues such as local pride, public transport and parking.
- Forget the politics. Councillors and MPs are key stakeholders and need special attention.

This requirement for collaboration may frustrate some GP commissioners who are keen to starting making a difference right away. But it is important to understand that the changes ultimately made will be all the stronger for public involvement. That is why ongoing dialogue with patients and public is more effective than ad hoc consultation. The NHS needs to make more of the resource that is already there. Foundation Trusts have huge ready-made focus groups through their thousands of members. Patient Participation Groups in general practice have developed into a useful network of engaged, informed people who want to contribute. In Nottinghamshire, a chance remark by a PPG member led to a county-wide campaign on missed GP appointments; research by the PCT revealed the clinical time being wasted across the year was the equivalent of six full time doctors or nurses.

Longer-term relationships are more productive because they are based on mutual understanding. Often, the most useful insights are gained not when reaction is being sought to a plan or idea, but when people are asked much more open questions. Both managers and clinicians often refer to patients attending A & E "inappropriately" – in the sense that the physical treatment required could have been provided elsewhere. But a mother with a feverish child will feel their visit to A & E is perfectly justified, because her primary motivation is reassurance. The only way to find that out is to ask her.

So clinicians should not be nervous about entering into conversation with the public. After all, they already have dialogue with their patients. This is about information – providing it, receiving it, and using it to improve things. Information is power. In his landmark report, Sir Michael Marmot (2010) concluded that the empowerment of individuals and communities would help to reduce health inequalities. The NHS Alliance goes further:

> ...empowerment for patients, service users and citizens also requires... a focus on supporting the delivery of personalised information that aims to elicit behaviour change. Information should increasingly be regarded as a 'therapy' in its own right, alongside drugs, surgery and other such interventions. (p6)

The most powerful example of empowerment through information has to be the Expert Patient Programme, where patients with long term conditions are trained to offer mutual support. Attending EPP groups can be an inspiring experience. Take the case of 67-year-old Geoff, a former miner who was diagnosed with chronic obstructive pulmonary disease:

> All of a sudden I realised I was getting my control back. I could do what I wanted to do. From a person who cried at night because he was desperate to die, I'm now a person who at night time plans what he's going to do tomorrow. We've all heard about glasses being half full or half empty. When I came from home from that Expert Patients group, my glass was brimming. I hadn't felt like that for years. I had a new life given back to me.

That is why hundreds of thousands of people work for the National Health Service, to help create more stories like Geoff's. There are times when we need hi-tech operating theatres and the best surgeons in the world. At other times, all we need is a helping hand. Through personalised care from clinicians who will forever be the glue in the system, the NHS can continue to give us what we need.

We need to change the relationship the health service has with the public and patients, to one of "co-production", so we can do the *Right Things*, safely and effectively. This will not only deliver what our patients need but will also help us to manage the relentless demand for healthcare within our available resources.

■ REFERENCES

Abbott, A. (1988). *The System of Professions*. An Essay on the Divisions of Expert Labour. Chicago: University of Chicago Press.

Ackoff, R L. (1994). *The Democratic Corporation*. New York: Oxford University Press.

Antropus, S. and Kitson, A. (1999) *Nursing Leadership: Influencing and shaping health policy and nursing practice*. Journal of Advanced Nursing, 29(3): 746-753. (Available at: www.journalofadvancednursing.com/docs/1365-2648.1999.00945.x.pdf)

Ayer, A. J. (1935) Language, Truth and Logic. Penguin,

Beattie A (1995). *War and peace among the health tribes*. In Soothill, K., MacKay, l., Webb, C. (Eds). Interprofessional Relations in Health Care (pp. 11–26). London: Edward Arnold.

Berwick D (1996) A primer on leading the improvement of systems BMJ 312 : 619

Boyle, D. and Harris, M. (2009) *"The Challenges of Co-Production"* 2009 NESTA http://www.nesta.org.uk/library/documents/Co-production-report.pdf

Brambleby P (2010) Third Annual Population Review www.rightcare.nhs.uk

Brigato & Jacobs (2003) Integrated Care Pathway Users Scotland (ICPUS). (2007) A Workbook for People Starting to Develop Integrated Care Pathways. ICPUS. (pp.6-7).

Brook R Managed Care Is Not the Problem, Quality Is JAMA. 1997;278(19):1612-1614.

Brooks R (2010) The End of the Quality Improvement Movement – long live improving value 2010;304(16):1831-1832. doi: 10.1001/jama.2010.1555

Burns, J. (1978) *Leadership*. New York: Harper Row.

Cabinet Office (2005) *Code of Practice on Consultation*. London: Crown copyright. (Available at: www.bis.gov.uk/assets/biscore/corporate/migratedd/publications/f/file47158.pdf)

Child, J. (2005) Organization. Contemporary Principles and Practice. Blackwell Publishing. (p.15).

Clay, S and Longman, H (2010) *Transformation of Urgent Care: How Evidence-Based GP Practice is Reducing Emergency Admission*. Presented at the NHS East Midlands Innovation Expo. (Available at: www.rightcare.nhs.uk/resources/index.html)

Cochrane AL. *Effectiveness and Efficiency*. Random Reflections on Health Services. London: Nuffield Provincial Hospitals Trust, 1972. (Reprinted in 1989 in association with the BMJ, Reprinted in 1999 for Nuffield Trust by the Royal Society of Medicine Press, London

Cyert, R.M & March, J.G. (1963) *Behavioral Theory of the Firm*. New Jersey: Prentice-Hall.

Daren, T. *et al*. (2008) Effect of financial incentives in the delivery of primary care in England. Lancet, 372: 728-736.

Dennis P (2007) Lean Production Simplified. A plan language guide to the world's most powerful production system. Productivity Press, New York. (p.15).

Department of Health (2008) *Real Involvement*. London: Crown copyright.

Department of Health. (2010) Equity and Excellence: Liberating the NHS. White Paper.

Donabedian, A. (1966) Evaluating the Quality of Medical Care. Millbank Memorial Fund Quarterly. 44: 166-203.

Donabedian A (2003) An introduction to quality assurance in healthcare :Oxford University Press

Drucker, P. (1955) The Practice of Management. Elsevier, Butterworth-Heinemann. (p.54-5).

Dusheiko, M., Gravelle, H., Jacobs, R., Smith, P. (2003) *The effect of budgets on doctor behaviour: evidence from a natural experiment*. CHE Technical Paper Series 26, University of York.

Easton J 2011 QIPP can provide 'crisis' needed to break hospital dependence www.hsj.co.uk/news/finance/easton-qipp

Elwyn, G. (2006) Developing a quality criteria framework for patient decision aids; online international Delphi Consensus process. BMJ, 333: 417-427.

Enthoven A & Smith K (2005) *How Much Is Enough?* Shaping the Defense Program, 1961-1969

Fisher C (2007)   Resource Allocation in the Public Sector *Values, priorities and markets in the management of public services* Routledge London

Freidson, E. (1984). The Changing Nature of Professional Control. *Annual Review Sociology*, 10, 1-20.

Gabe J *et al* (1991) The Sociology of the Health Service Routledge New York

Goldberg, D. and Huxley, P. (1980) Mental Illness in the Community: the Pathway to Psychiatric Care. UK: Tavistock Publications Ltd.

Gray, M. (cited 2011) *Doing the right things for patients*. Published via the Public Health Commissioning Network. (Available at: www.phcn.nhs.uk/Right%20care%20-%204.%20Doing%20the%20right%20things%20for%20patients.pdf).

Gray, M. (cited 2011) *How to get better value by doing the right things*. Published via the Public Health Commissioning Network. (Available at: www.phcn.nhs.uk/Right%20care%20-%204.%20Doing%20the%20right%20things%20for%20patients.pdf).

Hayek FA. (2009) The Use of Knowledge in Society. Library of Economics and Liberty.www.econlog.econlib.org/cgi-bin/printarticle.pl sourced on 10/11/209

Helman, C. (2002) *The Culture of General Practice*. British Journal of General Practice, 52(481): 619–620.

Hickson *et al.* (2007) Use of probiotic *Lactobacillus* preparation to prevent diarrhoea associated with antibiotics: randomised double blind controlled trial. Brit. Med. J. 335: 80-88.

Homa, P. (2011) *Communication Drives Change*. Health Service Journal, 21 April 2011.

Ipsos MORI (2010) *Commentary Report for the GP Patient Survey*. (Available at: www.gp-patient.co.uk/results/annual/commentary/)

Integrated Care Pathway Users Scotland (ICPUS). (2007) A Workbook for People Starting to Develop Integrated Care Pathways. ICPUS. (pp.6-7).

Kippist L (2004) The Paradoxical Role of the Hybrid Clinician Manager, Industry and Innovation Studies Group, University of Western Sydney, Penrith South 1797, NSW, Australia. l.kippist@uws.edu.au

Klien R (2006) The new politics of the NHS from creation to reinvention 5th edition Oxon Radcliffe

Kübler-Ross, E. (1969) *On Death and Dying*. New York: Macmillan.

Le Grand, J. (2007) The Other Invisible Hand: Delivering Public Services through Choice and Competition. USA and UK. New Jersey and Woodstock, Oxfordshire, 167-8.

Mandel, K.G. (2010) Aligning resources with large scale improvement. JAMA, 303: 663-4.

Marmot, Sir M. (2010) *Fair society, Healthy Lives*. (Available at: www.marmotreview.org).

Marshall, M. *et al* (2002) *A qualitative study of the cultural changes in primary care organisations needed to implement clinical governance*. British Journal of General Practice, 52(481): 641-645.

Mitton, C. and Donaldson, C. (2004) Priority setting toolkit. A guide to the use of economics in healthcare decision making. BMJ Publishing Group. (p.18)

Mooney, G.H., Russell, E.M., Weir, R.D. (1980) Choices for Health Care. Macmillan Press Ltd. (pp.10-11).

NHS Confederation (2008) *Principles for Accountability.* (Available at: www.nhsconfed.org/Publications/reports/Pages/Principlesforaccountability.aspx).

NHS Institute for Innovation & Improvement (online) *Clinical Engagement.* (Available at: www.institute.nhs.uk/quality_and_service_improvement_tools/quality_and_service_improvement_tools/clinical_engagement.html)

NHS Institute for Innovation & Improvement (online) *Experience Based Design.* (Available at: www.institute.nhs.uk/quality_and_value/experienced_based_design/the_ebd_approach_(experience_based_design).html)

Newhouse J (1992) Medical Care Costs: How much welfare is lost? Journal of Economic Perspectives, Vol6, No3,Summer 1992 (p3-21)

O'Connor, A. (cited 2011). Interviewed online at: www.rightcare.nhs.uk/presentations/index.html.

Oliver, S. (2006) *Leadership in health care.* Musculoskeletal Care, 4(1): 38–47.

Parry, K. and Proctor-Thomson, S. (2003) *Leadership, culture and performance: the case of the New Zealand public sector.* Journal of Change Management 3(4): 376-399.

Perrow, C. (1970) Organizational Analysis: a sociological view. Tavistock Publications, London.

Picker Institute (cited 2011) www.pickereurope.org/decisionsupport

Smythe, J. (2007) The CEO: *The Chief Engagement Officer.* Aldershot: Gower Publishing.

Porter ME. (2008) What is Value in Health Care? Harvard Business School. Institute for Strategy and Competitiveness. White Paper.

Porter ME Tiesberg EO:2006 Redefining Health Care: creating value based competition on results. Boston Harvard School

Porter ME (2010) What Is Value in Health Care? NEJM | December 8, 2010 | Topics: Cost of Health Care, Quality of Care

Rice, T. (1998) The Economics of Health Reconsidered. Health Administration Press, Chicago (pp.19-20).

Rowe J (2006) Pay-for-Performance and Accountability: Related Themes in Improving Health Care *Ann Intern Med.* 2006;145:695-699.

Scrivens, E. (2005) Quality, Risk and Control in health Care. Open University Press (p.91).

Stanton, E (2010) *et al* ; Clinical Leadership: Bridging the Divide London; Quay Books:2010

The Guardian (April 2011) *Open letter from the Federation of Surgical Specialty Associations.* (Available at: www.guardian.co.uk/society/2011/apr/18/open-letter-federation-surgical).

The NHS Alliance (2010). *Whose NHS Is it Anyway?* (Available at: www.nationalvoices.org.uk/sites/default/files/Whose_NHS_is_it_anyway.pdf).

Tsourapas A, Frew E (2011) Evaluating 'success' in programme budgeting and marginal analysis: a literature review *J Health Serv Res Policy* 2011;16:177-183 doi:10.1258/jhsrp.2010.009053

Valderas, J.M., Alonso, J. (2008) Patient reported outcome measures: a model-based classification system for research and clinical practice. Qual. Life. Res., 2008;17:1125. DOI 10.1007/s1136-008-9396-4. Accepted: 6 September 2008/Published online: 3 October 2008.

Walshe K (2010) Reorganisation of the NHS in England *BMJ* 2010;341:c3843

Wennberg, J.H. (2010) Time to tackle unwarranted variations in practice *BMJ* 2011; 342:d1513 BMJ 2011; 342:d1513

Wennberg, J. (cited 2011). Interviewed online at: www.rightcare.nhs.uk/presentations/index.html.

Woodard,F. (2007) *How to Achieve Effective Clinical Engagement and Leadership when Working Across Organisational Boundaries.* Guy's and St Thomas' Charity. (Available at: www.gsttcharity.org.uk/pdfs/mipracticalrecommendations.pdf).

Williams, S. (2004) *Evidence of the contribution leadership development for professional groups makes in driving their organisations forward.* Henley Management College, for the NHS Leadership Centre. (Available at: www.nursingleadership.org.uk/publications/LitRProfGps04%20(Henley).pdf)